Healing Plants

An Introduction to the healing power of plants

All rights reserved. No part of this publication may be reproduced or transmitted in any form or by any means, electronic or mechanical, including photocopy, recording, or any information storage and retrieval system, without permission in writing from the publisher.

Contents

Introduction 8
Chapter 1 – Historical Uses of Flowers and Plants 10
    Healthcare 12
    The Power of Aroma 13
    Prehistoric Times 14
    Ancient Egypt 15
    Incense 16
    Aromatic Oils 17
    Tribal Remedies and Plant Usage 19
    Other Ancient Remedies and Foods 21
    Biblical Plants 22
    Middle Ages 23
    Mandrake 26
    The Present Day 27
Chapter 2 – Health, Beauty and Cosmetics 28
    Bach Flower Remedies 28
    Aromatherapy 36
    Making Your Own Fragrance Oils 46
    Herbal and Homeopathic remedies 46
    Chinese Herbalism 58
    Creating the Right Atmosphere with Herbs 58
    Homoeopathy 58
    Making Your Own Cosmetics 60
        Cold Cream 60

A Moisturiser 61

A Toner 61

A Deodorant 62

A Face Pack 62

A Cleanser 63

A Facial Herbal Steam treatment 64

A Hair Tint 65

A Bath Treatment 66

A Skin Revitaliser with Fruit 66

Chapter 3 – Flowers and Meditation 68

Learning to relax 68

Creative Visualisation 72

Getting Started on a Visualisation 73

Meditation with a Flower 74

Meditation with a Journey 76

Other Meditations 79

Chapter 4 – Looking at Colour 82

The Importance of Colour 82

Colour and Health 83

Aura-Soma 84

Red 86

Orange 86

Yellow 87

Green 88

Blue 88

Indigo 89

Violet 89

Colour in Our Food 90

Colour in the Home 91

Chapter 5 – The Healing Garden 93

Making a Herbal Garden 93

Lesser-known Herbs 96

Drying and Storing Herbs 99

Drying Flowers and Making Potpourri 101

Scented Pillows 103

Plants for Your Garden 104

Eating Your Flowers 105

Thinking of Seasonal Garden Colours 106

Creating Single Colour Schemes 108

Small Garden Ideas 109

Chapter 6 – Plants and Flowers for Decoration 111

Buying House Plants 111

Talking to Plants 111

Colour in Plants 112

Looking After Cut Flowers 113

Prolonging the Life of an Arrangement 115

Flower Arrangements in the Home 116

Giving Gifts 117

Using Flowers in Decoration 118

Location, Design and Balance 118

Objects for Flower Arrangements..123

Introduction

In this book, we are going to take a look at what plants and herbs can do for us, to improve our health and our general wellbeing, including how to make various cosmetics using plants and herbs. We will learn how flowers can be used in meditations, how the use of colour affects us all, and how we can use fresh and dried flowers as decorations and for healing.

For centuries people have been aware that plants and flowers can be used in a healing capacity. Herbalism and homoeopathy, for example, are just two fields of therapy which use the inherent properties of plants and flowers to benefit health. Aromatherapy is another holistic therapy which seeks to reduce stress, illness and disease using the power of oils obtained from plants and flowers. The use of the power of flowers in healing is nothing new: the ancient Greeks used specific fragrances as healers, such as white violet for curing stomach upsets. Before the benefits of aromatherapy became widely known as an aid to relieving stress, scented bath cubes or various colognes or rosewaters were added to bathwater, not only to make the skin smell nice, but also to help the relaxation process.

Many people are now turning to the power of aroma therapy oils to achieve physical benefits and to address many psychological conditions which are now, sadly, commonplace in our lives. The Bach Flower Remedies (Bach is pronounced *batch*) help to heal us mentally and physically, so we will also take a look at these, and at the linking of oils and colours in Aura-Soma. We will discover the benefits of natural products over artificial substitutes.

If we can understand and appreciate what is around us in the world of flowers, perhaps we might be encouraged to protect flowers and plants for future generations. Many people are now actively engaged in fighting the development of urban areas in areas of outstanding natural beauty, and while not wishing to debate the rights and wrongs of what humankind seems to be doing to our planet, I believe that if we all understand a little more about nature, we will not seek to destroy so much of it so readily. Let's begin our journey of discovery, therefore, and take a more detailed look at the power of flowers.

Chapter 1 – Historical Uses of Flowers and Plants

Flowers, and also whole plants, barks, roots and herbs, have traditionally been used for a variety of things - not only for decorative purposes and gifts, but also in medicine, as fragrances, in skin and beauty preparations, and as food or decoration for food. In history, we used flowers and plants a little more in health care than is the case today, partly because many of the plants and (lowers held to be useful medically in the past may no longer have therapeutic value, due to interventions by medical science and technology. There are many plants, however, whose usage remains important. Mistletoe, for example, is known to be effective in treating high blood pressure and migraine, because it contains the drug guipsine. It has also been used effectively in the treatment of arteriosclerosis, and its Celtic name uile translates as 'all-healer'. Those suffering from dandruff might also like to try it in shampoo form, as it certainly works!
In this chapter, we will look at how our ancestors used (lowers, plants, herbs, shrubs and barks, for a variety of everyday uses, including medicine and beauty preparations. We will also consider the plants and flowers mentioned in the Bible - the word 'paradise' is derived from the Persian word for a walled garden!

Beauty and Healthcare

When you were a child at school, I am sure that one of the first topics you studied in History was the growth of and development of the human race. I remember learning about Troglodytes (cave dwellers) and visiting a museum where there was a 'mock-up' cave, complete with inhabitants, then subsequently going on a nature ramble with a teacher to look at the types of berries and plants that these cave dwellers probably used in their daily lives. I learnt, for example, that chewing on the leaves of a willow would cure a headache. This was a folk remedy from ancient times, which worked because the leaves of the willow contain a small portion of salicylic acid, which is a component of aspirin. It didn't taste too good, but it worked!

Beauty preparations

At school we also learnt a little about how other generations used various flowers and plants for beauty care. I remember vividly, when I was probably only about 8 years old, collecting what seemed at the time to be tonnes of rose petals to make some rosewater to use in the bath. Rosewater is useful in skincare preparations because it helps to soothe the skin and is a mild astringent. It is, incidentally, often used in commercial skincare preparations as a toner for those with dry skins. In the seventeenth century in Britain, women used rhubarb juice and white wine as a lightener for their hair and also used a mixture of burnt rosemary and alum flowers for cleaning their teeth - gruesome! Civilisations in the distant past used plants and flowers to help to improve their appearance, both by face painting and by using flowers as decorations, and also used flower oils as fragrance.

We still use flowers and their properties in skincare and beauty preparations. Many readers will be familiar with henna in shampoos and hair care preparations. Henna, particularly important in Muslim countries, is an evergreen shrub that has fragrant clusters of small cream coloured, four-petal flowers at the tips of each branch, and henna seeds have long been used to tint and dye the hair, finger and toe nails, fingertips, hands, feet, beards and even the manes, hoofs and tails of horses, as well as skins and leather. Many ancient Egyptian mummies appear to have been wrapped in cloth dyed with henna. Also, it is mentioned in the Bible in the Song of Solomon, and for many centuries, especially in the Middle East, henna's strong fragrance has been popular. Many Eastern races use henna in bouquets, and women wear it in their hair and put it on their clothing. Other natural hair and body dyes and tints can be obtained from camomile, marigold flowers, saffron roots or flowers, turmeric, rhubarb (also a good laxative) and sage (good to use in the bath), but more of that later.

Healthcare

Saffron is also mentioned in the Bible in the Song of Solomon. An Old World crocus, it takes about 4,000 blooms to make just 28 grams (1 oz) of saffron, using the dried styles and stigmas of the flowers. Consequently, saffron is quite expensive to use, but makes a lovely herbal tea beneficial in treating skin or liver problems, and is a good flavouring for foods. It was also formerly used as a perfume. Another flower mentioned in the Bible is the lily, which Jesus mentions in the Gospels according to Matthew and Luke. In Biblical terms, the lily and beauty were interchangeable. The marshmallow plant, closely related to the hollyhock, is mentioned in the Bible in Job as being used as food in times of hardship. Its tastelessness was obviously a strong point in its favour, as many other plants were known to have a bitter taste. Nowadays used as an ingredient of facepacks, it can also be used in the form of a tea for treating digestive problems, especially in children.

The ancient Greeks used a great number of plants for health benefits. Plants were used in drinks, and a trip to any health store or supermarket will reveal many plant-based teas now available.

The ancient Greeks, Romans and Egyptians used juniper berries in medicine, and in later medieval times, these berries were considered to be remedies for ailments as diverse as snake bites and the plague, while in Tibetan history various species of juniper are claimed to be useful in cancer treatments.

Hippocrates, from whom comes the Hippocratic Oath which doctors take, is known to have used plants in his treatments, including many quite common flowers and fruits. Likewise, Galen, personal doctor to many Roman emperors, used plants and flowers in his healing work, and his copious records are well worth reading. Incidentally, cold cream, still used by many as a beauty preparation and skincare aid, was invented by Galen.

Many tribes of the world still use the plant life around them for their remedies. Many of us in the Western world have lost the desire or abilities we perhaps all once had to produce remedies for ourselves; we have become reliant upon others for this help. Although there are those in our societies, the shamans, medicine men, healers or health care workers, whose primary aim in life is to help us to feel better about ourselves and find a way of conquering those ailments which beset us, we also need to rediscover how we can open ourselves up to other avenues where, with a little time, knowledge, patience and effort, we can help ourselves to make our own preparations. A little later in this book, we will talk about making such preparations, and how various flowers and plants can help us to improve our lives and our health. We should, however, take care with herbal medicines, and should consider consulting a qualified herbal practitioner. In the meantime, it is worth remembering that we all use natural remedies, albeit rarely. For example, most of us will know that dock leaves, growing by the side of stinging nettles, are a treatment for the sting of the nettle, as well as being useful for combating other skin rashes. Many plants and flowers are poisonous, and it is important to be able to distinguish these, not only for medicinal use, but equally for food.

The Power of Aroma

We can be attracted to flowers by their colour, by their form and by their smell. Scientists suggest that 17,000 smells, good, bad and indifferent, have been distinguished, and even psychiatrists will sometimes use the power of smell to bring out deap-seated memories in patients. Smell has probably been one of our most used senses, and one of the most powerful, since early times.

Prehistoric Times

Early humans probably used the sense of smell primarily to distinguish whether a substance was good to eat or not. Relying on taste as a first resort is not always advisable! When gathered around their fires in their caves, early humans probably became used to the differing smells of burning woods. They would have discovered that some woods, when burnt, gave off soothing fragrances, while others were less pleasant. Certain woods may have been observed to give people heightened experiences, and as a result, many peoples concluded that the smoke of the fires held some magical or mystical properties. Laurel was often burnt in religious ceremonies by the priestesses at Delphi as a means of creating prophetic visions. A similar tradition still exists in India and Java, where priests regularly inhale aromatic smoke before making prophecies. Likewise in various Voodoo traditions in Haiti, perfume and magic are closely linked. In Western culture, some groups believed that a mixture of sandalwood, hemlock and coriander could, when burnt, summon up demons. If henbane was added, this would enhance the experience.

Most cave people would have had little knowledge of what their bodies were like internally, other than what they might have assumed from cutting up animals for food. Their use of natural substances, of plants and flowers, was the result of many experiments. Their knowledge of burning different woods developed into using fragrances to both hide other smells, to soothe or allure, for beauty purposes and to heal. They probably also began to realise that certain berries, roots and leaves when ingested made people feel better, and that animals also ate natural substances when ill in order to make themselves better. The beneficial effects of aromas and fragrances has not been confined to humans. It is well known amongst country folk that dogs can be calmed by a mixture of the copaiba, aniseed and rhodium fragrances, and that horses will generally respond better to a handler who has around him or her the smell of fennel

Ancient Egypt

It is uncertain when the use of fragrances for health benefits really began, although the use of fragrances in ancient Egypt was widespread, and it is known that frankincense, for example, was used in 3500 BCE (Before Common Era) by the priestesses in the temples. The ancient Egyptians believed that the gods lived in the fragrance and petals of flowers, and often laid floral tributes on or near the altars of their gods. Ra, the Sun god, was often portrayed surrounded by volumes of flowers, and statues to him were crowned with flowers, woven together. The volume of flowers used was considered a significant factor, and thus many statues were literally surrounded by flower offerings. In some cases, however, a certain flower was associated with a particular god, and only one kind of flower would be offered. The ancient Egyptians used the flower known as the everlasting flower in their tributes to the Sun god, possibly because of the flower's ability to last a long time, and flowers were carried in the processions at the annual Festival of Shrines. It is interesting to relate this to the use of flowers within churches around the world today. Flowers are still used to decorate altars, and at times, such as Harvest Festival, other plants and wild flowers are brought into the churches. The original pagan tradition of linking flowers and candles is worthy of note, as not only candles are used to mark important celebrations, but also flowers. The ancient Egyptians also used perfumes and flowers to mark funeral occasions, and many oils were used in funeral tributes. It is said that a sealed alabaster vase discovered in 1922 when the excavations of Tutankhamen's tomb took place still gave off a mild fragrance.

Incense

The use of incense and fragrance was once widespread. One of the earliest recorded incense formulas appears in the Bible in Exodus 30:34 where the holy incense of the Israelites is described. One of the main items carried by the caravans of Oriental traders who journeyed the spice routes to Damascus is pure frankincense, a sweetly scented substance, much like gum, which comes from certain trees in India and Arabia. Frankincense is still used widely in religious ceremonies, and is a great aid to meditation when used in oil form in an aroma therapy vaporiser or as an incense. Valued and prized as highly as precious jewels to the ancient Egyptians, frankincense was often used to aid concentration, alleviate toothache and breathing problems and cleanse wounds.

One can only assume that the medicinal benefits of various plants and herbs came about due to much experimentation. People would pass on their knowledge to those within their communities, and such knowledge would then spread. To the Babylonians, flowers, herbs, roots and trees were often used in prescriptions for health benefits, and clay tablets still survive with Sumerian notations upon them, listing such things. The Babylonians as a race were less disposed to be accurate with their writings, and we do not have details of the actual quantities used or the exact formulae. However, we do know that an ancient Babylonian king had within his garden most of the plants which are today actively used within herbalism and aroma therapy.

Within ancient Egypt, those who dealt in the sale of fragrances were important, as it is recorded that certain young men used up to 15 different types of fragrances to attract women. For their part, the women hid globules of aromatic substances in their hair. The use of incense was also extensive and sophisticated, and most incenses are made of a single substance, rather than a mixture, so that each can be more accurately reproduced at a future time.

Aromatic Oils

The Romans also used fragrances, especially aromatic herbs, within their homes and daily lives. The Romans used marjoram for their hair, mint for an underarm deodorant and palm oil as an aftershave. Within the ancient Roman, Greek and Egyptian civilisations anointing oils were used not only in religious ceremonies but also by others for the fragrance emitted and also for medicinal value. Anointing oils are still sometimes used, especially for coronations, and Queen Victoria is said to have disliked the smell of the original coronation oil to such an extreme that another, more acceptable, fragrance was developed. This formula is still used at such occasions.

It is supposed that much of the information for using plants in healthcare came from the Greeks. It is well documented that the Greeks used olive oil to absorb the fragrances of various flowers, so that the perfumed oil resulting could be used for either healthcare purposes or in beauty preparations. It is also recorded that Greek soldiers would carry ointment made from myrrh into battle to help in the healing of wounds. Myrrh comes from an Israeli shrub with fragrant wood and bark. It is known to help with mouth and throat infections and can be useful as a tonic to improve a jaded appetite. Myrrh is said to symbolise the suffering of Christ, and was known in the time of Cleopatra to be useful as a skin preservative, hence its use in embalming the Egyptian dead.

Another well-used plant is rosemary, mentioned in Shakespeare's *Hamlet* as being 'for remembrance'. The Greeks used rosemary both in cooking and at shrines where it was burnt, it was sacred to the Romans, and it was used throughout the Middle Ages in exorcisms and in sickrooms as a means of reducing disease. Rosemary has strong antiseptic properties, can help with respiratory problems, can delay putrefaction in meat, can hide underlying bad tastes and is also a brain stimulant. It can also be used in hair care preparations, especially for those with dark hair, and is said to help bring back colour to greying hair. It is also one of the original ingredients of eau de Cologne.

In China, the tradition of herbal medicine and using plants, flowers and barks in healing goes back to before 2000 BCE. The Chinese herbal medicine classic known as Pen ts'ao kang-mou lists over 8,000 different formulae, many using plants, as well as minerals, and it is recorded that, as long ago as 1000 BCE, the Chinese used opium for the treatment of dysentery.

The Chinese left records going back over 4,000 years detailing many herbal remedies. One remedy, based on the juice of a Chinese fir tree, Ma Huang, was said to cure bronchitis and asthma, and research on this remedy carried out in 1878, found that the juice contains the alkaloid ephedrine, which became used in the treatment of pulmonary disorders, eases breathing, especially in cases of asthma, and is also useful in cases of hay fever. Herbal cures still feature strongly in Chinese healthcare, and there are many herbal dispensaries in their hospitals. Likewise in India, the Ayurvedic medical practitioners (from two Sanskrit words 'ayur' meaning life and 'veda' meaning knowledge) use herbs in their cures and remedies, as well as vegetables and minerals.

The Romans, more interested in simple things which could be prepared themselves at home, were well versed in the use of flowers and plants, and were very successful in the field of preventive medicine, using natural substances to prevent an illness from becoming serious.

The Bible details several plants and flowers used in the preparation of food and culinary matters. Mint, dill, cumin, rue and mustard leaves were all actively used, and the caper berry was used as an appetiser. The pods of the carob tree were usually fed to animals, young vine leaves were eaten as a green vegetable, the root of the broom tree was eaten, and endive and chicory were used at times of Passover. Manna, which was probably coriander seeds, was the basic food for the Israelites when in the wilderness, and was ground into cakes. The peoples of that time also used plants and fruits for medical care, and it is known that fig poultices were often used. Galen, who was born in Asia Minor (now Turkey) around 131 CE, learnt a great deal about the body from treating gladiators' wounds with plant and flower remedies.

In Arabia just prior to 1000 CE a Persian doctor, Avicenna, used plants and herbs for health benefits and left details of over 800 plants and their effects, which has been most useful for those following on. Avicenna also discovered how to distil the essential oils which are used in aromatherapy.

Tribal Remedies and Plant Usage

Many primitive peoples had knowledge of plants and their healing abilities, and this has been passed down to our present day in manyof the remaining indigenous tribes of the world without ever having been formally recorded.

Many South American plants and herbs are now actively used within health care. Statistics suggest that around 80 % of the world's herbal flora can be found within the Amazon basin and an American University has been experimenting with more than 1,000 of these plants for many years, knowing that for centuries the Indians of the Amazon have been using them in healthcare. It is known, for example, that certain tribes will use the bark from a willow tree, infuse it in boiling water, and drink it when they have headaches. Likewise, digitalis which comes from the common purple foxglove was used by many tribes in South America for heart problems, and it is common knowledge that digitalis can reduce the pulse rate and also promote the secretion of urine. As such, herbalists such as George Graves, who wrote *Hortus Medicus* in 1834 recommended its use, with care, for inflammatory conditions of the chest as well as for palpitations and other ailments.

Cures for coughs, colds, skin complaints and rheumatism are all actively made from plants, flowers and roots. Quinine is a commonly used medicine which was first used by the Indians of South America.

Within the culture of the North American Indians herbal, flower and plant remedies abounded. It is known that the Dakota tribe relieved asthma with the powdered roots of skunk cabbage, that the Kiowas used a plant called soap root in the treatment of dandruff and that the Cheyennes would drink a tonic of boiled wild mint when nauseous. Other Indian remedies included black nightshade, which was a Comanche tuberculosis remedy, Indian turnip which was a Pawnee headache remedy and yarrow, which was used by the Utes for healing cuts and bruises. The Crees were known to chew on the tiny cones of spruce trees to soothe sore throats, and many frontiersmen owe their lives to the remedies given to them by friendly Indians. It is said that Prince Maximillian's life was saved in 1834 by an Indian remedy of eating raw bulbs of wild garlic. In recognition of the medicinal value of Indian cures, the authoritative US Pharmacopoeia and the National Formulary officially accepted 170 Indian natural remedies.

Other Ancient Remedies and Foods

For centuries plants and flowers have been used worldwide for cooking and in the preparation and presentation of food. We still use mint in cooking and in confectionery. Mint can aid digestion, it can also help at the start of a cold, and in certain cases some forms of mint can be useful for headaches, flatulence, insomnia and nausea. Parsley is used as a tonic and also a diuretic. Not only is parsley a medicinal plant, but it is also a culinary herb. Garlic is also used in cooking and in capsule form for its health benefits. In Egyptian times gangs of slaves, who were used to build the pyramids, were given a daily ration of garlic as it was known to help prevent the infections and fevers prevalent at that time. Garlic is now recognised as a digestive stimulant, an antibiotic and an antispasmodic.

In ancient Egypt records were made of the herbs, flowers and plants used by priests and healers and their benefits were thus preserved. In fact, one papyrus said to date back to 1500 BCE lists literally hundreds of herbal remedies, many used in the daily diet, as can be said of the use of garlic. The earliest papyrus recording the use of plants for medicinal purposes dates from around 2890 BCE. It listed not only which plants were used but also trees, roots, bulbs, herbs, fruits and vegetables. As well as providing minerals and vitamins, these herbs and flowers also added a great deal to both the taste and presentation of food. The nasturtium plant is still used in salads to add to the taste of what can otherwise be a bland meal. I must admit that I particularly like nasturtium leaves and have used them many times in salads much to the amusement and amazement of visitors. I have also eaten the dried flowers of the marigold in soups, broths and stews, and found that they add a lot to the flavour. They can also be used in salads and can help with indigestion and gall bladder disorders, as well as being used within cosmetics in creams for chapped hands and chilblains. Marigold oil is also used to soften the skin and soothe irritation.

The North American Indians used a wide variety of plants in their foods. Sweet thistle stalks were peeled and were said to taste like bananas. Milkweed buds and rosehips were used, along with the sliced fruit of the prickly-pear cactus and added to soups and stews.

Wild fruits and a great variety of roots and stalks were also used for culinary purposes. Not a people likely to waste anything which could be used, vegetables and fruits were often stored in large jug shaped caches dug into the ground.

Biblical Plants

There are several types of plants and flowers mentioned in the Bible, including the vine and the olive tree. The word of Gethsemane (as in Garden of Gethsemane) means 'oil press'. The vine is important for producing grapes and is mentioned throughout the Bible from Genesis onwards. Likewise the olive tree is important as it is able to grow in poor soil, yields a rich supply of fat in the form of olive oil and can be used for cooking, lighting, cosmetics and medicinal purposes. Olives were pickled in brine and stored, and provided year round nourishment. In Palestine in the spring, wherever cultivation is not too intensive and wild plants are allowed to grow unhindered, a carpet of colour spreads across the countryside prior to the summer drought, with different flowers appearing and fading away in rapid succession. Poppies, camomile, corn marigold, wild anemone, cyclamen and more come and go in waves of colour. Lilies, mentioned by Jesus in Matthew 6:28-30 ('consider the lilies of the field) how they grow; they neither toil nor spin, and yet I say to you that even Solomon in all his glory was not arrayed like one of these') were probably one of the more global 'lilies of the field' such as poppies. Earlier in the scriptures in Isaiah 40:6-8, we read 'All men are like grass, and all their glory is like the flowers of the field. The grass withers and the flowers fall, but the word of God stands forever'. Most people in Biblical times lived in rural areas and were intimately aware of the natural world around them. They realised that their lives depended on agriculture and when plants and herbs were mentioned in the scriptures, even as illustrations and as metaphors, the people understood the underlying meaning. Mustard is mentioned in Matthew 13:31-2 where it is compared to the Kingdom of Heaven. In Biblical times, mustard was used both as a cooking oil and for medicinal purposes in the making of poultices or plasters. Wormwood is mentioned in Revelation 8: 10-11, where following the sounding by the third angel, 'a third of the waters became wormwood'. Wormwood is a herb which can grow up to a metre in height and is often used to stimulate the digestive system. In the Bible the plant's bitterness is always stressed - it also has a sickly smell and Proverbs also mentions at 5:4 that 'her end is bitter as wormwood'.

Middle Ages

We know that during the time of the Crusades many knights brought back spices, herbs and fragrances from their travels. They learnt how to distil perfumes and the use of more European flowers, such as lavender, became commonplace. Many trained to become apothecaries, herbalists and health workers. Between 400 and 1000 CE the growth of use of herbs was immense. In the 9th century, a medical school opened in Salerno in Italy, which specialised in herbal cures. Many respected scholars came to the school, including Constantinus, a translator from Africa, who translated medical books from Arabic into Latin, enabling many to learn about herbal remedies used in the Middle East.

In the 12th century, the first perfume manufacturers emerged, and lavender water was one of the most popular fragrances. In Italy the manufacture of lavender water became central to the economy, especially during the Renaissance, but later France became the place where the majority of lavender waters and perfumes were made.

Many monasteries in the Middle Ages specialised in treating illness, and as such herbs and plants were grown in the monastery grounds. As the plants were grown on holy soil, it was thought that the resultant healing would be of religious significance, and God was given the credit for the healing.

It was noticed at an early stage that poppy juice could make people drowsy, and the juices were given either in a mixture or on a piece of cloth, their fumes inhaled in order to perform operations more successfully. It is interesting to note that Sornnus, the ancient God of sleep had the poppy as his flower and it was used as a tribute and placed around statues.

Those interested in Shakespeare might already know that many flowers were mentioned in the various plays. The gillyflower is mentioned in *The Winter's Tale,* the cowslip in *A Midsummer Night's Dream,* and pansies and rosemary in *Hamlet.* Another prominent plant used at the time was the deadly nightshade. Witches throughout medieval Europe used the plant in their spells and ointments as the whole plant is poisonous due to the presence of alkaloids like hyoscyamine. Mentioned in *Macbeth,* where it was used to knock out the invading Danes, eye drops were, and still are, sometimes made from belladonna and in many homoeopathic preparations, belladonna is used to great effect.

In medieval times people believed that fragrances could protect people from illness and save people from plagues. Around this time, the British rhyme *Ring O' Roses* was first heard and the line 'A pocketful of posies, a tichoo a tichoo, we all fall down' reminds us that people carried bundles of flowers to protect their health. From the 1700s, ladies regularly used to carry pomanders of flower heads within their clothing to give off a pleasant aroma, and flowers and herbs were strewn around the

floors of buildings to protect people from infection, especially during the times of plague and pestilence.
Although considered to be more superstition by many, it is now known that such things have the ability to repel insects and act as disinfectants. During the Black Death (1348-1349) doctors, who stayed in the cities to treat people, put on gowns and hoods with beaks, which they stuffed with herbs or with sponges soaked in vinegar in an attempt to remain free from illness. Oranges, stuffed with cloves, were used as pomanders and records tell of huge bonfires on which herbs were burned to clear the air of the smell of disease. Even in Victorian times, it was quite common to spray tube rose in the room or parlour where a coffin was being kept prior to the funeral. As few people could afford a doctor herbal homemade remedies were much used. Occasionally, the visit of 'a travelling bonesetter' would help the sick and ill, but herbal and flower remedies were more widely available and were obtained from the gardens in the neighbourhood or by roadsides.

Nicholas Culpeper, the 17th century doctor, actively supported the use of common plants and flowers in his treatments, which are detailed in his celebrated book *The English Physician Enlarged*, written in 1649. Some of his treatments might now be considered a little unsuitable - for example he suggested that the berries of the hollybush could be used to expel wind and treat colic, and that the bark and leaves, when fermented, were good for treating broken bones. Culpeper also considered mistletoe berries to be useful, especially for treating headaches. Like Culpeper, Gerard and Banckes in England, Nicolas Monardes in Spain and Otto Brunfels, Leonard Fuchs and Hieronymus Bock in Germany made great inroads into the study of plants.

With advances in printing of the written word around the 15th century, various books and journals became available to the public listing herbal remedies. For example John Parkinson of London listed over 3,000 useful plant remedies in his book of

1630. Likewise, Mattioli's herbal, written slightly earlier, was translated into several languages, and sold over 32,000 copies in the 16th century.

Mandrake

Mandrake was popular in the Middle Ages for treating insomnia. For those who are unfamiliar with mandrake, it is common in many countries and is related to the potato. In England a version of the black bryony plant was often substituted for mandrake, and in the time of Henry VII, this false mandrake was used in assisting birth. Mandrake is mentioned in the Bible in Genesis 30: 14 where we are told that Reuben went and found mandrake, gave them to his mother, Leah, and she conceived a fifth son. In ancient times mandrake was used as a narcotic and antispasmodic and is still used in the Middle East as an aphrodisiac and fertility aid. The peoples of that time were most particular how the plant should be gathered. As the roots fork, it was felt to be symbolic of the human body and was thought to shriek in pain when pulled from the earth, illustrated by Shakespeare's play, *Romeo and Juliet*, where Juliet feared 'shrieks like mandrakes torn out of the earth'. If pulled by its roots it was said that the person responsible would go mad or die. As a result, the roots were gathered with care at sunset. String was attached close to the roots, while the other end was tied round the neck of a hungry dog. Meat was thrown in front of the dog so that it was unable to reach the meat without pulling up the mandrake plant, thus the plant was pulled up by something other than human hand.

Mandrake appears in early Greek herbal remedies and was dedicated to Hecate, Greek goddess of magic and the darker side of things. Found in Tutankhamun's tomb, the Arabs called the fruits of the mandrake Satan's Apples. Used widely in ancient times as an anaesthetic, mandrake could ward off pain and promote sleep if used in small quantities, and was interestingly one of the remedies stocked in the drugstores of the towns of the Wild West, along with squaw vine and summer savory, although most of the remedies sold at such drugstores relied heavily on their alcohol content to work.

The Present Day

Plant and flower-based therapies, from herbalism and aromatherapy through to the Bach Flower Remedies are readily available at many health shop outlets. Scientific advances, however, have lead to a decline in the usage of herbal and natural remedies, even though *Potters Cyclopaedia of Botanical Drugs and Preparations* has never been out of print since it was published in 1812. Fortunately, over the last couple of decades, the speed of this decline has lessened, with more and more people becoming aware of the potential of flowers, plants, herbs and shrubs. Various tests, trials and investigations into the medicinal properties of plants continues to take place, and organisations are continually being set up to study this field. Many people, concerned about the possible side effects of taking mass-produced chemicals have taken to herbal and natural remedies, citing that they offer a safer and more effective treatment.

Chapter 2 – Health, Beauty and Cosmetics

We are now going to look at how plants and flowers are used in our modem age. When we think of flowers and plants in connection with health there are a couple of therapies which may spring to mind immediately - Bach Flower Remedies and aroma therapy. During the course of this chapter, we will consider both of these and other treatments where flowers and plants may be enlisted to aid us, in addition to learning how to make our own beauty preparations.

Bach Flower Remedies

Edward Bach's remedies, based on 38 preparations made from wild flowers and plants, are now readily available all over the world.

Edward Bach (1880-1936) was a notable physician and bacteriologist who qualified at University College London and subsequently gained his diploma in Public Health at Cambridge before beginning his career in 1915. A consultant at a leading London hospital and author of several highly-respected medical papers, Edward Bach practiced, very successfully, in London's Harley Street, home of many eminent doctors, but even as a student he was far more interested in patients as people rather than in mere diseases. He quickly began to realise that people's emotional and mental state played a large part in the rate at which they recovered from illnesses and observed early on in his career that patients needed to overcome negative thinking if they were to return to good health.

In 1917, Edward Bach fell ill. Whilst working at University College Hospital in London, he collapsed and suffered a severe haemorrhage. Told that he had some rare disease and only three months to live, Bach wanted to continue to find remedies to help his patients, and toiled hard looking for a cure. He believed that most drugs were frequently ineffective and possibly even dangerous, and that allopathy simply suppressed symptoms without getting to the root causes of the illness. He discovered, as a result of his work, that he could use plants for the treatment of illnesses and concentrated his attention on which illnesses they could cure. Bach made a miraculous recovery himself, not only living considerably longer than the three months he had been given, but going on to enjoy better health than he had previously enjoyed.

In 1930, convinced of his theories, Bach abandoned his Harley Street practice and moved to Wales where he continued to research the healing properties of plants. Discovering mimulus (for any disease whose root cause was fear) and impatiens (for impatient people), the first two of his remedies, he set to work on discovering a further 36.

Bach's interest in homoeopathy and knowledge about the work of Hahnernann, the founder of homoeopathy, helped him in his work. He used to walk miles each day through the Welsh countryside getting to know the plants and wild flowers, looking at whether they seemed to enjoy sunshine or prefer shade. He theorised that the dew on the flower heads could contain the full properties of the plant, and discovered that the dew collected from flowers growing in shady places was less potent than that of flowers exposed to sunshine, thus reinforcing an ancient belief that the sun itself has healing properties. He found that the most effective way of obtaining a plant's properties was by placing the flower heads in a clear glass bowl of spring water and standing it for several hours in the place where the plants grew. He was so concerned that the flower heads remained untouched after this process that he lifted them from the solution with a blade of grass.

After publishers rejected his work he went to stay in Cromer, and it was here that he discovered the 12 wild flowers which he was to use as remedies. One experiment on agrimony saw a middle-aged alcoholic woman, who previously had been unable to eat or sleep and who drank throughout the day, improving to the stage where, after five weeks, she was eating and sleeping, and drinking only in moderation. Bach subsequently went to Eastbourne, discovering the gorse, oak and heather remedies and the Rescue Remedy, about which more later.

Bach intended his remedies to be so simple that anybody could use them, without having to consult a professional therapist. He suggested that an illness should not be viewed in isolation but as with homoeopathy, the whole character, mental attitude and emotions of the patient should be considered so that the treatment is truly holistic (that is covering the whole person, not just the illness). His resultant 38 remedies based on negative mental states became known as Bach Flower Remedies, after his name, and as they are homoeopathically prepared, they can be taken by anybody with complete confidence. They have no side effects and do not react unfavourably with any other drugs, homoeopathic or allopathic.

Dr Bach identified seven different types of negative emotion and the plants which alleviate them. These states of mind are: apprehension and fear; uncertainty and indecision; loneliness; apathy and lack of interest; oversensitivity to influence and ideas; despondency and despair and finally excessive concern for the welfare of others. Bach believed that prolonged states of mental negativity would result in a loss of vitality and a weakened physical body making it easier for viral infections to invade the body. Bach demonstrated that once a state of peace and tranquillity were restored to the mind by using his remedies, the body would set about healing itself. Bach suffered many setbacks in trying to get his remedies accepted and available. Magazines were generally unwilling to print his advertisements and when finally successful he became the subject of much criticism from the General Medical Council. Bach continued practicing the remedies up until his death in

1936, having dedicated his whole life to the alleviation of emotional and physical pain.

Bach's remedies are so gentle in action that, not only are they safe to use with children and pets, but it is necessary to take them for several weeks before real results become apparent. One of the few remedies where this does not apply is the Rescue Remedy, which can help immediately in cases of acute distress, mental upset or shock. The Rescue Remedy will also help combat stresses which are known to be just around the corner, and which could lead to a state of imbalance or anxiety, such as if you are taking a driving test, speaking in public, or an important business meeting. It can also help with cases of insomnia because of its calmative properties. Containing the flowers of rock rose (extreme fear), clematis (confusion), impatiens (mental stress), cherry plum (desperation) and star of Bethlehem (for cases of shock), I have used this on many occasions with good results and it is extremely valuable in all first-aid situations. It is available in liquid form and in a cream, which can be used on stings, cuts and abrasions. If you come across someone in need of this remedy, you might consider placing a little behind the ears or on the insides of the wrists, rather than trying to get the person concerned to take some orally. Alternatively, you can use the remedy on cotton wool pads in the form of a compress.

Bach's 38 remedies and their uses are listed below but it is worthwhile pointing out that there is much more information available on these remedies than has been possible to give here, and interested readers would do well to contact the Dr Edward Bach Centre, at Mount Vernon, Sotwell, Wallingford, Oxfordshire, OX10 0PZ. Before embarking on using these remedies it is important to make sure that you look at all the salient mental characteristics of the person concerned. You may need help assessing your own characteristics as it is difficult to look at ourselves objectively. Only a couple of drops of each remedy are needed in a cup of clean water, with food. The remedy is generally drunk four times a day for a couple of weeks at the very least. In emergency situations the remedies can be used to moisten the lips, gums or tongue until signs of recovery are evident, particularly so in the case of the Rescue Remedy.

Agrimony
Helps with inner turmoil or torment, hidden worries and anxieties which cannot be shared, leading to stress. Self-torture behind a cheerful face.

Aspen
Combats fears which cannot be accounted for. Anxiety for no apparent reason, with an inability to even voice the problem. Feelings of apprehension.

Beech
Useful for those overly critical, dogmatic persons with intolerance towards other people's shortcomings. These people need to learn to be more tolerant towards the shortcomings they envisage they see in themselves and in others.

Centaury
For those always concerned with pleasing others and too gentle for their own good, so that they are often put upon by others. Easily lead and exploited.

Cerato
Helps those lacking in self-confidence, always seeking approval and advice from others. Doubting own judgement and capabilities, and so always asking others to make even the simplest of decisions for them.

Cherry plum
For fear of losing control and doing something wrong. Fearful of being unable to resist impulses, tension, despair, desperation, fear and irrational thoughts.

Chestnut bud
Helps the person who doesn't learn by previous mistakes, so makes the same mistakes over and over again. Mistrusts advice of others.

Chicory

Offers help to the over possessive, those with a degree of self-praise, who cannot bear to let those whom they love live their own lives. Clinging, bossy, mothering types.

Clematis

Help for daydreamers, indifferent to others, idealistic, quiet and unhappy. These are escapists and often absent minded and mentally confused. When ill, these people lack the energy and resolve to regain their health.

Crab apple

For those fearing something is amiss, feels shame at ailments or general self-disgust, this is a general all-round healer and natural purifier.

Elm

Help for those suffering from inadequacy, incompetence and striving for the impossible, suitable for those with overwhelming responsibilities.

Gentian

If feeling discouraged and feeling loss of heart, this remedy offers encouragement to those who feel that things are too great to overcome.

Gorse

Good in cases of hopelessness, despair, helplessness, feeling everything has been tried and nothing more can be done. Pessimism and defeat.

Heather

For those who are confident and capable, good at advising others and very competent, but impatient and expecting others to act as promptly as they personally do. Self-centred, talkative about self and past experiences.

Holly

Combats envy, hatred, jealousy, revenge, suspicion and negativity which prevents fulfilling relationships by being totally negative and potentially destructive.

Honeysuckle

Help for those who are suffering from dominant nostalgia, living in the past, yearning for what might have been instead of facing up to situations. Homesickness.

Hornbeam
Good for mental and physical exhaustion, feeling unable to cope, however misplaced this feeling may be, the 'Monday morning feeling', procrastination.

Impatiens
A remedy for impatience, tension, irritability, good for stress. This remedy will help whether the impatience is aimed at the person concerned or somebody else, or indeed with life generally.

Larch
These are the people who are lacking in confidence and think of failure, feelings of inferiority, lack of self-confidence, and don't even try.

Mimulus
Helps with fears of an unknown origin, and a real comforter in the problems and fears of everyday life, shyness, timidity, dread of illness, pain or accident, loneliness, poverty and the loss of something or someone dear.

Mustard
For depression which comes and goes, but is often severe. Feeling overwhelmed by a dark cloud, and feeling sad and low for no apparent reason. This remedy will help restore balance and lift spirits.

Oak
If you refuse to give in, but feel hopeless, this is the remedy for you. People who struggle with any adversity, when all is against them, naturally strong and tenacious, but need a bit of extra help.

Olive
Useful if suffering from temporary shock, physical or mental exhaustion, or feels that someone is 'having a go' at them over a period of time.

Pine
People who blame themselves for the mistakes of others, who feel guilty for their own inadequacies, and those who always apologise benefit from this remedy. Never content with their own efforts or results.

Red chestnut
A combat for those who worry excessively for others and feel that something dreadful will befall them, especially so if the other person is someone close. Caring but overly concerned.
Rock rose
For extreme panic, fear or fright, due to something unexpected, sudden illness, bad news concerning self or a loved one.
Rock water
This is for the martyrs, who subjugate their own personal happiness for others or for work concerns without thought for its effects on others.
Scleranthus
For people who cannot make up their minds, never make a positive decision, change like the wind and suffer from fluctuating moods and vacillation.
Star of Bethlehem
Great for mental, emotional or physical shock, such as following serious news, a traumatic experience or a fright following an accident or attack of any kind.
Sweet chestnut
Useful in cases of despair, bleak outlook, dejection and mental anguish.
Vervain
For those who are over-tense, nervous, strong-willed and courageous, who keep going until they collapse. Over-enthusiastic or with fanatical beliefs.
Vine
A remedy for the totally dominant and completely rigid person. Ambitious, inflexible, tyrannical, arrogant, autocratic, bossy, these people cannot accept help from others at all, even when it is willingly given and needed, because they are never wrong.
Walnut
For help needed with change, either in circumstances or in health, particularly useful at menopause and puberty. For those concerned with other people's view of life. Oversensitive people who always take into account the ideas and opinions of others and need to let go.

Water violet
A remedy for aloof, proud people, who are determined to get on with their own lives even though there may be inner doubts. Like being alone. Reserved.

White chestnut
For people who have difficulty concentrating or keeping fixed, so mentally wonder and fritter energies away on trivialities. Mental conflict. Good to help those who want to meditate but find it hard.

Wild oat
For those who suffer from dissatisfaction but are unable to do anything about it and unsure of which direction to take in life. Good when the patient fails to respond to other treatments. Uplifting and calming for troubled nerves.

Wild rose
For feelings of apathy, feeling everything is too much trouble, despondency without a cause. Resigned to situations, even if not happy with them.

Willow
For those suffering from despair and embitterment because of misfortune, but not able to face up to the realities of the situation. Someone who continually moans about their lot in life.

Bach Flower Remedies are extremely effective, totally natural and without side effects. If you feel any of the remedies listed above could possibly help you, do try them because you have nothing to lose, and a lot to gain.

Aromatherapy

Aromatherapy is a potent treatment which uses flowers to combat stress, stress-related illnesses and many other physical ailments. Aromatherapists use what in medieval times became known as the doctrine of Signatures - this suggests that the shape, aroma or colour of a plant gives an idea of the qualities that the plant possesses, and by learning to read this Signature you can find out which plant to use for which disorder.

Throughout history many people have successfully used aromatherapy and its essential oils to treat various illnesses and afflictions. The Ancient Egyptians used aromatic oils not only for religious purposes, but also in massage, perfumery and embalmment. As we have learnt, pomanders made of oranges, herbs and spices were popular in the time of the plague to ward off illness. Culpeper, who we also mentioned in connection with his herbal research, used amongst others the essential oils of peppermint and rosemary in his work. However, it is not until the 20th century that the term aromatherapy was coined - by a Frenchman called Rene Gatefosse, who was working in a laboratory of a perfumery when he badly burnt his hand. Access to water was limited, but nearby was a bowl containing essential oil of lavender. Gatefosse observed that the hand healed quickly and left little scarring and realised that the qualities of the pure essential oil of lavender were greater than those of commercially mass-produced substances. As a result of this incident, he researched essential oils in depth and he published his first book of aromatherapy in 1928. His research was supplemented by Dr Jean Valnet, another Frenchman, who worked as a medical surgeon during the Second World War at a time when medical supplies were difficult to obtain. He used essential oils to treat various battle injuries and he later treated his patients in a psychiatric hospital with the oils and other plant and flower products with great success. His book *The Practice of Aromatherapy* became one of the foremost books on the subject. Aromatherapy, like Bach Flower Remedies, not only seeks to treat an illness but also helps the mental state of the patient thus offering a holistic experience.

Oils can be used in massage, in the bath, inhalation, for compresses, for creating a pleasant smell in a room and for helping in the recovery from illness. I have successfully used aromatherpay oils around the home, despite not having a sense of smell myself, by using vaporisers, by putting spots of oil on light fittings, on radiators and by spraying into the room in cases of illness.

Clinical trials at the Kneipp Institute in Germany have shown that essential oils are absorbed by the skin, enter the bloodstream and can be measured in the exhaled breath. In much the same way, the smell of the oils also affects the body and those who scoff at this idea would do well to remember the effects of glue sniffing, anaesthetics or cigarette smoke to realise that there is a definite link between what we breathe in and our state of mind and health. Used as a complement to other therapies, as well as being a therapy in its own right, aroma therapists have to undergo a great deal of training and recognised qualifications can be obtained. The International Federation of Aromatherapists sets high standards in its examinations and trains many people from all over the world.

Aromatherapy oils can be made from many different parts of a plant: from flower, seed, fruit, leaf, root or wood, in the case of trees. Most oils are made from a distillation process and various parts of the same plant or tree can be used to produce different oils. Some flowers are too fragile to cope with the distillation process so a solvent extraction process is adopted. This is a long process and often results in the oils being costly to produce. However, one only has to smell the oil of jasmine, which is made by the solvent extraction process, to realise that this is really a small price to pay for such a wonderful oil.

Aromatherapy oils are widely available at various outlets but I would give one word of caution here. There is a wealth of difference between a pure essential oil and a fragrance oil. Fragrance oils are normally chemically based and are simulations of a natural smell. They are great to use in potpourris and the like but should not be confused with essential oils'. Also be careful when you buy oils that call themselves 'aromatherapy oils' as some of these may not have pure essential oil in them. Make sure you buy the best quality oils, and price can often be a guide, although it is not unheard of for unscrupulous traders to pitch a chemically-based oil at a higher price to deliberately confuse.

Neat essential oils should never be used directly on the skin, with the exception of lavender oil, and should never be ingested. Be very careful when using on babies and children, and in cases of pregnancy avoid oils which are stimulating or which can help to bring on periods. Similarly, if you are using homoeopathic remedies check whether the oils will nullify the homoeopathic preparations. It is recommended that the interested reader should seek out a book specially dedicated to the art of aroma therapy.

Blending mixtures of your own oils is a great experience, and even the novice should experiment a little. As a general rule you shouldn't blend more than three oils together although there are exceptions such as lavender oil which will blend with lots of other oils.

Aromatherapy oils should be stored in dark bottles away from the light with the bottle tops tightly screwed. Most essential oils will, if kept properly, last for up to two years.

Aromatherapy oils can be divided into three categories - top, middle or base notes - depending on their rate of evaporation. The top note makes the initial impact, the middle note provides the mellow fragrance, whilst the base note is the lasting fragrance. If you wish to blend oils, you need a carrier oil. I recommend sweet almond oil, because of its vitamin E content, and its easy absorption. Others might think in terms of grape seed. To mix an aroma therapy massage oil, use just 20-30 drops of essential oil in enough carrier oil for the finished product to fill a 2 fluid ounce bottle. Massage the area gently and remember that a teaspoonful is enough to treat a whole back, so use it sparingly. If possible use circular motions using the fingers as well as the palm of the hand.

If you wish to try a compress, 10 drops of oil to half a cup of water will be enough. Soak your cotton wool or bandage well, wring it out, wrap around the affected area and then cover with Clingfilm.

If you wish to use aromatherapy oils in the bath, use 6 or 8 drops and make sure that you stay in the bath for at least 10 minutes to reap the benefit. In the case of footbaths or hand baths, 10 drops of essential oil in a bowl of hand-hot water will serve the purpose. For many centuries, the healing powers of water therapy (hydrotherapy) have been known and spas, saunas and whirlpools are now quite common in health clubs, leisure centres and also in some homes.
Even Hippocrates acknowledged that 'the way to health is to have an aromatic bath and scented massage every day.' For women who have just had babies, or for people with genito-urinary infections, hip baths or sitz baths using essential oils can help greatly with the healing processes. For inhalation purposes, a few drops of your chosen oil on a handkerchief, in a vaporiser or on pillowcase will usually be enough.

For general skin care it is possible to use aromatherapy oils sparingly in prepared skincare products and creams. Lavender, neroli and patchouli, for example, will help rejuvenate the skin and neroli, sandalwood and cypress can be used on sensitive skins as a treatment for broken veins. If you wish to try this out, just add a few drops to a previously fragrance free day cream. We will discuss other beauty preparations using plants and flowers in a later chapter.

There is a wide variety of aromatherapy oils now available for use, and what follows is only a selection. I have indicated which should not be used by pregnant women, and which are suitable for young children.

Basil
Great for nervous problems, for uplifting the spirits, chest infections, headaches, sinus problems, listlessness and depression. Can be used in cases of fainting or in exam situations, but not for pregnant women. If blended with lavender, this oil is great for overtired muscles and is especially useful for dancers and athletes.

Benzoin

A resin, an ingredient of incense and one of the components of 'Friars Balsam', it is great for chest infections, arthritis, blisters, chilblains and tension, due to its relaxing and warming properties. It is also good to use when feeling down as it helps to lift the spirits.

Bergamot
One of the most popular oils, coming from the orange, it helps greatly with PMT, depression, lack of motivation and stress, ulcers, chickenpox, vitiligo, cystitis, sore throats and psoriasis. This oil should not be used if a person is likely to be going into the sun or onto a sunbed within three hours of application as it is phototoxic, and skin pigmentation can be affected. Bergamot, incidentally, is the flavour of Earl Grey tea, and can help to regulate the appetite.

Black pepper
One of the oldest oils, this is great for aches and pains, flu symptoms, digestive problems and catarrh. A great stimulator, and if used in very small quantities with rosemary oil in a carrier base, it has proven to be useful for athletes, dancers and marathon runners, whose performance is said to improve and who suffer less muscular pain and fatigue after exercise. Be careful with this oil as too much can cause irritation.

Cedarwood
Used by the Egyptians in their mummification processes, for cosmetics and as an insect repellent, this oil will help with stress and anxiety, coughs, colds, asthma, and also dandruff when

added to a shampoo. This oil should not be used by pregnant women. It is also great for urinary tract infections.

Clary sage
This is 'the' PMT oil. It has properties which help relax the muscles, and is great for high blood pressure, menstrual problems, insomnia, exhaustion, as well as overwork and hyperactivity. Good to relax in the bath with, but should not be used by expectant mothers.

Cypress
Made from the leaves and cones of the cypress tree, this is an oil which helps with varicose veins, menopausal problems, makes an excellent foot bath, helps with asthma and coughs, haemorrhoids and, it is said, helps with cellulite.

Eucalyptus
Another ancient oil, this is one of the best natural antiseptics going and it is great for coughs, colds, bronchial problems, catarrh, congestion and sinus problems, as it helps to clear the head and relax the muscles. These relaxant properties make it a good massage oil for muscular sprains. This is a strong oil and should be used sparingly. Try spraying this in the sickroom or in a compress to reduce high temperatures, or mix with lemon and tea tree oil to make a great cold remedy.

Fennel
This oil will help with flatulence, indigestion, nausea and was traditionally used to help with obesity. It is said that Roman soldiers carried fennel with them to chew during marches when they had no time to eat. It can help with stomach pains, kidney stones, gout and toxic build-up if gently massaged in a carrier oil on the area concerned. It is also useful for menopausal women and is a natural diuretic. It is particularly effective if mixed with juniper oil. This oil should not be used by pregnant women or by those with sensitive skins.

Frankincense
Relaxing, spicy, warm and highly prized by many ancient cultures, this oil will help with colds, is an aid to meditation, is good in cases of nerves, panic attacks and nightmares, and is useful in cases of cystitis, heavy periods and skin problems.

Great for stress, this is one oil which should feature in most people's collection of oils as it can help combat fears and lift those who are down.

Geranium
Refreshing and relaxing, this oil stimulates the lymphatic system, blends well, and is great for skin problems, cellulite treatments, urinary disorders and viral infections. Used by many women around the menopause, it helps to balance the hormones, and can also be used in pregnancy to relax and relieve depression. Known to help with hormone problems, this is another oil used in PMT treatment.

Jasmine
One of the most expensive oils, jasmine makes a great massage oil when used in childbirth and will also help in flu cases.
It is useful in cases of apathy, lethargy and sadness, and this uplifting oil can also help with skin problems. Jasmine is popular with those with strong opinions - and people who make their minds up on new acquaintances immediately.

Lavender
Most people will have this oil in their first aid aromatherapy kit. It is useful for so many things, from skin problems and arthritis through to menopausal difficulties, migraines, tension, PMT, pregnancy, sunburn and earache. This oil, which works well in massage, will also help lift spirits especially after illness, aid relaxation and restful sleep, and is often used by theatricals in cases of stage fright or nerves, particularly if the stomach is likely to be affected. Lavender, when mixed with ylang ylang in the bath, makes for a wonderful relaxant, and it is interesting that the word 'lavender' comes from *lavare* to wash. Lavender was extremely popular with the Romans and is the safest of all aroma therapy oils, and as such it is great to use on children. It is said that lavender is generally popular amongst those who are conventional and unreceptive to new ideas.

Lemon
Great to use on warts, I have even successfully used it on animals to clear such things, as well as using it effectively on

acne, boils, corns and verrucae. This oil will help with circulation problems, and should be massaged upwards.

Marjoram

Not to be used by pregnant women, this oil is good for bruises, cramps and sports injuries, will relax the muscles and ease stress. As it has sedative properties it can also be used in cases of migraine, high blood pressure and insomnia, but for this reason should be used sparingly.

Myrrh

Another ancient oil, this is great to use in cases of dry coughs and colds, as well as in cases of mouth ulcers, thrush and catarrh. This was one of the oils Greek soldiers carried into battle to treat their wounds.

Neroli

I use this oil regularly in a carrier base as a facial oil as it helps stimulate the growth of new cells. It is also worth trying on stretch marks and scars. One of the ingredients of a true eau-decologne, this is also useful in cases of stress, bereavement or shock and aids restful sleep. This oil is known as orange blossom.

Patchouli

Musky and traditional, this oil, which is one of the few which improves with age, is often used in the perfume industry. Relaxing and calming, it help with mental clarity, lifts depression, and is great on skin problems and wounds, especially athlete's foot, when used in a carrier base. This is an oil you will either love or hate, and another which is thought to have aphrodisiac properties.

Peppermint

Used widely for digestive problems by many people, not just those interested in aromatherapy, peppermint is also good to relax in the bath with at the end of a hard day used sparingly – one drop in a bath is sufficient - it is great for bilious attacks, headaches, migraine, nausea and travel sickness. A compress using peppermint can help with mastitis. Should not be used by expectant mothers.

Roseotto

Great for PMT, migraine, hangovers and hay fever, it will also help with depression, nerves, fright and grief, and can be useful in creams for mature skins (just a drop in a jar is enough). The Greeks thought that white rose oil used in a house would create a harmonious atmosphere in which love overcame all fears. Rose as a smell is usually liked by those who are sincere in affection and of an intense nature. It is popular for use on children.

Rosemary
Put a couple of drops of rosemary oil on your clothing and feel better. This oil will help clear the head, get rid of sluggishness, tiredness and overexertion. It is useful in a carrier base for treating sports injuries and is popular with marathon runners. Known to be good for circulation problems and great as a tonic for oily skin, rosemary will also help with colds, bronchitis and flu symptoms. It should not be used by pregnant women.

Sandalwood
Used for centuries in India for medicinal use, this oil is good for colds, coughs, sore throats, bronchitis, loss of voice, sinus problems and hoarseness, and can also help lift spirits and help with nervous problems. Try it as a compress for shaving rashes. Popular with those who like to be different in any way.

Tea tree (also spelt as Ti-Tree)
Anti-bacterial, anti-fungal and a stimulant to the immune system, this popular oil, used extensively in Australia and by the Aborigines for centuries, contains substances not found elsewhere in nature. Known to help with colds, tonsillitis, acne, mouth alcers, verrucae, thrush and sore throats, this is another oil which can help if dropped onto the pillow at night. Try mixing it in a cream for warts, verrucae, corns and boils. You might also wish to try mixing it in a carrier oil for use on cold sores or sunburn or in a glass of water as a mouthwash for toothache.

Ylang ylang
This oil, whose name means 'Flower of Flowers', helps with nervous problems, builds confidence and lifts the spirits. Calming, soothing and relaxing, ylang ylang can slow down rapid

breathing caused by stress. Ylang ylang is popular with women and it is also said to have aphrodisiac qualities!

Making Your Own Fragrance Oils

If you wish to have a go at making some fragrant oils for yourself, all you need to get started is some fragrant flowers, a sterile glass jar with stopper, some cold-pressed sunflower oil and a small sieve. I would stress that the resulting oil will not be as intense or possibly as beneficial from a health angle as pure essential oil, but it is a great way of making the most of highly-scented flowers such as lavender or roses. Pick the flowers on the point of opening, and dry them on kitchen paper. Remove the petals from the flowers and pack as many of them as you possibly can into the jar. Pour in the oil, enough to cover the petals, and replace the stopper. Leave the jar outside in the sun for a few weeks, bringing it indoors at night. Strain through a sieve and discard the flowers. Repeat using the infusing process with more petals until the oil is sufficiently perfumed. Should you run out of petals, add a little pure essential oil to intensify the fragrance.

Herbal and Homeopathic remedies

Many people now take herbal remedies, normally in capsule form, to help their health and well-being. The benefit of herbal remedies lies in the fact that there are no side effects. However, because they are more gentle in action, the speed at which an illness or disease responds may be slower than with allopathic medicine. Many herbal remedies are now available in shops, but in days gone by, people prepared their own herbal remedies from the herbs which were available locally to them.

As we have already discovered, much of the current medical knowledge began with a knowledge of herbs and their uses.

Used for thousands of years in the treatment of illness, many herbal remedies have been passed down by families and records stretch back many centuries on trials and experiments undertaken by herbal practitioners. The *Ebers Papyrus,* written in 1550 BCE, for example, contains references to more than 700 herbal remedies, many of which are still used today. Likewise, details of herbal use in China goes back to the first century BCE and beyond. An ancient Ethiopian text, known as *The Book of Enoch,* written between the first and second centuries BCE, tells of the use of various herbs. Dioscorides, a Greek doctor, working with the Roman armies under Emperor Nero collected much information on medicinal plants and this textbooks were used for more than thirteen centuries. When the Romans came to Britain, they brought with them the knowledge of over 400 varieties of herbs plus many of the herbs themselves, including rosemary, sage, parsley and thyme. Later, in the time of James I, John Gerard, an English herbalist, published a book in 1597 describing about 2,000 different medicinal plants. As we have already mentioned, the most famous herbalist in history was probably Nicholas Culpeper, who worked long and hard to establish details on the medicinal values of herbs and plants and whose book, which was published in 1653 became essential to the study and use of herbs.

Not all herbal remedies come from ancient times. For example, the use of feverfew to prevent migraine attacks is a recent discovery: a doctor's wife, troubled by terrible migraine headaches, found conventional preparations ineffective. She was recommended by a local miner to chew the leaves of the feverfew, despite their bitter taste and she discovered the number and severity of the attacks began to lessen until, eventually after some time, she was more or less free of attacks. Her husband began to talk about this to colleagues and clinical tests were undertaken, some of which were published in *The Lancet* medical journal in July 1988.

Most herbal medicines use the whole plant *(totum)* and not just the flowers. This is due to a process known as synergism which is when two or more elements are used together to produce a greater effect. However, a branch of herbalism known as phytotherapy, from the Greek word for plant *(phyto)* and the word *therapy* meaning care, has gained popularity in the last few years. Using a capsule containing either the whole plant or the appropriate part, which has been ground up into a powder using laboratory skills, phytotherapy capsules have little taste, but the benefit of the plant or herb used will be the same as using the whole plant. Practitioners of phytotherapy would suggest that extracts and teas from plants may not be as effective but nevertheless many herbal remedies can still be made outside of laboratory conditions, although many require certain skills and experience. The preparation of herbal remedies can often involve much training and research. Medical herbalists regularly usecombinations of plants, and for complex medical problems it is strongly advised that a qualified, reputable medical herbalist be consulted. In Britain, the letters FNIMH or MNIMH after a name indicates extensive training and membership of the National Institute of Medical Herbalists. Many herbal remedies, which are available at health shops and through mail order are worth trying out but you are advised to seek further information on the herbs, especially if you are hoping to treat a serious or persistent problem.

Herbal teas or infusions are well worth trying out. There are many varieties, from teas which will help to combat colds (peppermint is one of these) to teas like camomile, which will help calm frayed nerves. To make an infusion, take one ounce of the dried or fresh flowers or leaves to one pint of boiling water, then strain and take in doses of two or three tablespoons at a time. You might also consider using a tisane, a milder version of an infusion, which are sold in teabags in most health stores. Make with boiling water, and drink more or less straight away. For a decoction, take one ounce of root, or powdered dried herb, boil in one pint of water using a stainless steel or enamel

saucepan (not aluminium), leave to stand until cool, strain and take in doses of one tablespoon at a time. If you wish to try a tincture, put about 4 ounces of ground or chopped herb into a container, add a pint of 40 % alcohol (gin or vodka are useful here) and seal the container. Leave in a warm, dry place for a couple of weeks, but make sure you shake the bottle at least twice a day. Decant the liquid into a dark wine bottle, seal and use when you need to. You can also use herbs in the form of a compress by using either a hot herbal decoction or an infusion as a poultice, by using fresh untreated herbs directly onto the skin, or by placing between a piece of gauze.
You can also use dried herbs and make a paste with hot water and apply to the skin. Herbal ingredients can also be added to creams and ointments and marigold ointment is very good for skin problems. You may also consider using herbal baths: the use of hydrotherapy with plants is not a new idea, and many people are now taking an interest in natural spring waters or spa towns, where the mineral contents of the water reacts favourably with herbal preparations.

Please remember that herbal treatments may take a time to help with an illness, after all most illnesses take a time to develop, and their severity will vary depending upon the patient and other factors. Some remedies suit a certain group of people more than others, and some illnesses are easily treated, whereas some may take longer to respond. We have tried to include as many and as wide a variety of herbs as possible in the following brief guide, but it is recommended that those readers interested in the application and uses of herbs consider further research, as it is not possible to list all the herbs.

Aloe vera
This cactus-like plant is used for a variety of purposes: from helping skin and hair problems through to maintenance of good intestinal health. Known as the 'medicinal plant', and used by the ancient Romans, Greeks, Chinese and Indians, it is widely available in health stores in many forms, including gels and

cosmetics, the latter being reputedly used by Cleopatra. The leaves of the plant contain a rich gel which is used in many other preparations, and is a good treatment in the event of sunburn.

Angelica
Used to treat coughs, colds and pleurisy, this is an ingredient of Vermouth and Chartreuse. Also used as a tonic, the root is the most active part, whilst the seeds are also sometimes used as carminatives.

Arnica
The flowers of this mountainous plant are useful in cases of depression and rheumatism and infusions are most popular. Also useful in skin care products, especially hand lotions.

Balm
Cures headaches, coughs and flu symptoms, and if used externally it makes a good insect repellent.

Basil
Helps with coughs and colds, bronchial complaints and digestive problems. It has been used to treat nervous headaches, and is sacred to Krishna and Vishnu in India because it is said to improve masculine vigour.

Belladonna
Otherwise known as deadly nightshade, it was used in the past to combat bladder spasms, coughs and asthma. The alkaloid atropine, which derived from belladonna, is a painkilling drug when used in small quantities.

Bergamot
This plant has lots of red tubular flowers, which are popular with bees. Growing to around 1.2 m, the leaves have a mint-like aroma and can be used in cooking and in aromatherapy.

Borage
Helps to alleviate melancholy but also used as a diuretic and as a cure for fevers and inflammation of the eyes. Borage is especially useful in cases of rheumatism and as a cough or cold treatment. This is a herb which most will find easy to grow and can be used in salads and in a tisane. Starflower oil, a derivative of the borage plant, has been shown to have beneficial effects

on the maintenance of a healthy skin. It is also claimed to help breast tenderness in women prior to their periods. Borage can also help in cases of stress and depression.
Broom
Useful in the treatment of bladder and kidney infections.
Celandine
Useful for treating warts, ringworm and haemorrhoids.
This plant was very popular in the Middle Ages. It was sometimes called swallow-wort because it was thought that swallows used the plant to cure myopia in their young, and it was thus used to treat eye problems. It was also thought that celandine was a cure for jaundice because of its yellow flowers.
Celery seed
This herbal extract helps maintain a healthy urinary system. It is worthwhile noting that commercially-produced celery seed capsules are likely to contain parsley seed, boldo extract, bladderwrack, kelp and alfalfa.
Cinchona bark
From this plant, the drug quinine is derived.
Chive
A natural antibiotic containing iron, oils, pectin and sulphur.
Colts foot Great for chest problems and often used as a component of cough medicines. It is now commonly used as an infusion to treat asthma and cases of influenza.
Cumin
This herb is a close relative of coriander, dill and fennel, and grows in the Mediterranean and Far East. Black cumin seed was especially revered by the Ancient Egyptians and is one of the ancient remedies presently undergoing many clinical tests worldwide. The oil from this seed is felt to have similar traits to evening primrose oil and it also contains properties which are felt to help stabilise the body's response to allergic stimuli. Cumin is also widely used as a general tonic and stimulant.
Dandelion
Dandelion is thought to be useful in cases of liver, urinary and skin problems. It has been used for centuries in Europe as a tonic due to its high iron content and is also used to treat

rheumatism, water retention and hypertension. The juice from the stem will help clear up warts, especially if aided by fresh lemon juice or crushed garlic. The root contains diuretic properties and various stimulants, and can be used to treat gallstones, dyspepsia and water retention.
Dock
This plant is not only an antidote to stinging nettles, which it grows near to, but is also useful for other skin rashes.
Elder
Much used for wine-making, the flowers of the elder are stimulating and useful for inflammation of the eyes. Elderflower lotions are often used to help make the skin soft and white, due to the presence of small quantities of ammonia within the flowers. An infusion of elderflower and peppermint taken three times per day can make a good cold remedy, helping to aid sleep and promote sweating. It is also useful in the treatment of strains.
Evening primrose
Introduced from America, the plant grows to around 80 cm, and has bright yellow, cup-shaped flowers. The oil from this plant can help with various women's problems, skin complaints and can help achieve a feeling of well-being.
Feverfew
A variety of the camomile plant feverfew is used to treat fevers, migraines and stomach upsets. If you wish to try this plant for migraine relief, either make an infusion or eat the leaves in a sandwich, preferably with something sweet to offset the bitter taste of the leaves. Feverfew tablets are also available from health stores. The plant is highly aromatic and is a wonderful asset to most gardens.
Foxglove
Used in the past as a treatment for weak hearts, this plant contains digitalis which has a specific effect on heart muscles and was also used to treat tuberculosis in the past. The painkiller digitalin is also derived from the foxglove.
Garlic

Garlic is useful for stomach problems, asthma and bronchitis, and much research continues into its curative properties, especially for cases of atherosclerosis, but it can also be used in either oil or capsule form to prevent colds and to help sinus problems. Used in cough syrups, it is also useful in lowering high blood pressure. You may also find garlic and parsley capsules help with digestive problems.

Germander
Used in the treatment of rheumatism and *gout:*

Ginseng
Popular in China and used for many years as a tonic, claims are presently being made about its aphrodisiac qualities, although this may be a fanciful thought! There are many types of ginseng available commercially, including Siberian, Manchurian and Korean ginseng. Combined with the Brazilian herb guarana, this herb has gained a lot of popularity with people looking for extra energy.

Hyssop
Used in the manufacture of liqueurs, the green tops were once used for stomach problems, chest infections and rheumatism.

Ivy
Both common ivy and ground ivy are used in cases of nausea, bums and scolds. Ivy leaves can be used as compresses and poultices for boils, skin problems, abscesses, and tired eyes. Ivy juice will help with colds and catarrh.

Juniper
Used widely in the treatment of back strain, rheumatism and liver problems. The berries are particularly useful as a diuretic and tonic.

Lemon balm
Useful to reduce the flow of blood when placed on an open wound. It is also said that lemon balm tea can help to prolong your life!

Loosestrife
In days gone by this herb was popular as a gargle for sore throats and was used to reduce the flow of blood from an open wound.

Lovage
Claims were once made that a lovage compress would clear freckles. Helpful in the treatment of stomach ache.
Male fern
The juice can help to eliminate tapeworm.
Mandrake
Common in Biblical times, this herb was used as a painkiller and sleep inducer.
Marigold
Useful in the treatment of eye infections, bee stings, depression and high temperatures. Marigold flowers can be added to broths, stews and salads and can be used in poultices and compresses for insect bites, skin inflammations, acne, burns and scalds, especially if combined with witchhazel. A tincture of marigold can be used to treat athlete's foot. Around an ounce of marigold flowers to a pint of boiling water will help in the treatment of cuts and abrasions. Calendula creams (marigold) are also used to treat cuts.
Marshmallow
Marshmallow is useful for bladder disorders and has, for centuries, been used as a component of cold lozenges in parts of Europe. The roots are useful as a poultice for bronchial problems.
Meadowsweet
Meadowsweet is good for treating diarrhoea and also useful for stomach upsets. An infusion of meadowsweet, ash and bog bean will help rheumatism and arthritic conditions, and an infusion of meadowsweet with cinnamon to taste, will help with vomiting. The distilled water from the flowers can be used in cases of fevers and eye infections.
Mint
This plant, especially wild mint, is useful for stomach upsets and will help with the digestive processes. In the 14th century, it was felt that eating mint would help to whiten the teeth. Culpeper suggested it as a remedy for sore mouth and gums. The variety of mint known as Pineapple Mint can be very refreshing and is worth seeking out.

Mistletoe
Once known as the 'cure all plant', mistletoe can be used for ailments as diverse as toothache and heart problems.
Motherwort
Useful in the treatment of 'women's problems' and anything relating to nervous tension.
Mugwort
Helps keep lethargy at bay. It is also said to help with poor eyesight when used as a poultice or in a tisane.
Nettle
Used for sore throats, gargles, mouth ulcers, high blood pressure and anaemia. As a diuretic it is often used, especially as an infusion, to help with fluid retention. A decoction of the root will help in cases of diarrhoea and it is still used to help stop nosebleeds. An infusion of nettles, strained into a bath of warm water, will help with backache, whilst a similar infusion in a footbath can help with gout. An infusion of equal parts of fresh nettles and rosemary to a pint of water will help with dandruff, hair loss or brittle hair if rubbed into a clean scalp and left for ten minutes. A similar treatment can be used for brittle nails.
Orris root
Useful in the treatment of bronchitis and dropsy.
Parsley
Commonly used in cooking, this herb can help with rheumatism and kidney problems.
Periwinkle
Chew this to help with toothache. It can also be taken to ease the pain of tight muscles or boils.
Peyote
Common in Mexico, this herb is widely used to combat hunger and thirst, and it also acts as an antidepressant and fear expellant! The narcotic mescalin is now known to be an active ingredient of this plant.
Poppies
Opium poppies are used to treat various illnesses due to the presence of morphine, heroin and codeine.

Primrose
Useful for coughs and colds, headaches, tension and stress. The roots can be used as an emetic. When mixed with' motherwort, it is helpful in the treatment of rheumatic complaints.

Quince
Used in ancient times as a cure against stomach problems. The mucilage from the seeds is still used in the treatment of dysentery and diarrhoea.

Rauwolfia
Used in the treatment of nervous disorders, high blood pressure and headaches. This plant has been found to contain various alkaloids, which are widely used today in medical practice.

Rosemary
It is said that rosemary will help with memory problems and dizziness. It is widely used today in hair tonics and shampoos to treat oily hair.

Sage
Used to help aching joints, depression, anxiety and headaches. In the form of a poultice, sage is used to cure sores and ulcers. Sage teas are useful for sore throats and as a tonic for the digestive and nervous systems.

Southernwood
Useful as an insect repellent.

St John's Wort
An ancient 'cure-all', said to help with wounds, stings and nausea. It is now more commonly used as a nerve tonic and painkiller. Combined with marshmallow, it can be used in skincare treatments. In cases of dizziness a little St John's wort oil held under the nose can bring a patient around. The patient will soon recover if this is combined with an infusion of peppermint tea. An infusion of 3-4 tablespoons of St John's wort can help people suffering from fatigue or mild cases of ME. St John's wort (also known as Pas siflora) can help with cases of chronic depression.

Tansy

Once used for sunburn, freckles and warts, it is now more commonly used for worms in children. It is also good for aching joints when made into a compress.

Thyme
This plant contains thymol, which is used for treating whooping cough.

Valerian
This plant is a mild tranquilliser and its root is commonly used in cases of nervous exhaustion. Most health stores sell relaxing herbal capsules, and it is usual to find that valerian is one of the ingredients. It should be pointed out that most herbalists will suggest that valerian be taken under their professional guidance, unless used as a tisane and taken in small quantities for a short time.

Vervain
In times gone by vervain was used in cases of swelling. Vervain is said to be useful for up to 30 different complaints and is now more often used as a cold remedy when combined with coltsfoot, as a treatment for diarrhoea or for stress-related illnesses.

White horehound
Helps the healing process when applied to cuts and bruises. It is also useful for coughs, colds and catarrh.

Wild strawberry
A good source of vitamin C and consequently useful as a tonic and as an aid for colds or flu.

Willow
Useful for its painkilling properties. Willow leaves and barks can also be used in malaria and dysentery treatments.

Wormwood
Used to help with digestion and as a tonic. Wormwood can also be used as a compress in the case of bruising to prevent discoloration of the skin. This herb is also used in the alcoholic drink absinthe.

Yarrow

Along with elderflower and peppermint, this herb can help lower blood pressure and speed up blood-clotting. It is also used for cold treatments.

Chinese Herbalism

Chinese herbalism is a very detailed practice which requires much skill. It includes within its framework herbal, animal and mineral remedies, breathing techniques and exercise, as well as dietary therapies. Based on Taoist philosophies, Chinese herbalism seeks to readjust imbalance within the body of Yin and Yang (the feminine and masculine) using the Ch'i or energy force. All organs are associated with the elements and are categorised as Yin or Yang. By using the pulses located in the wrist and by checking the skin, eyes, hair and tongue the Chinese herbalist will prescribe various herbs. Further reading is well advised as this is a complex subject and deserves far more space than we have available here.

Creating the Right Atmosphere with Herbs

Burning woody or resinous herbs can add a great deal to the atmosphere within the home. You can do this either over an open fire or by using a small incense burner filled with charcoal. Burning rosemary, for example, has an uplifting effect and helps clear and lighten the mind. Dried pine needles can also work well. Crushed carnations, ideally sun-dried, with a little carnation oil produces an energising atmosphere.

Homoeopathy

Akin to herbalism is the practice of homoeopathy. The term homoeopathy comes from Greek words *homoios* and *pathos* meaning 'like or same suffering'. Homoeopathy, then, is essentially the medical practice of treating like with like. It looks at the whole individual, takes into account lifestyle, attitude, emotions, likes and dislikes to help prescribe a treatment. Modern homoeopathy owes its prominence to the work of Dr Samuel Hahnemann, an early 19th century German physician. Hahnemann gave up his medical career in the late 1780s when he found himself totally disgusted at medical practices, which served to weaken the patient rather than improve overall health and strength. Hahnemann turned to translation to earn a living and when working on a herbal textbook he learnt that quinine, from chinchona bark, was good for malaria because it was a powerful astringent. Hahnemann took a healthy person, gave him a dose of the bark and found that it caused the patient to exhibit the symptoms of malaria. After realising that the patient's condition worsened before showing signs of improvement he went on to treat people suffering from malaria using diluted doses of the bark. He continued to research the ability of homoeopathy to stimulate the body's own immune system and produced a large amount of literature on homoeopathy, its proving (drug pictures) and results - his book *Der Organon* is still the basic homoeopathic textbook. Homoeopathy is a science and homoeopathic remedies, which can be used on children, adults and pets, should be prescribed by a qualified homoeopath. The selection of a suitable and appropriate treatment is important. There are, for example, over 50 different types of homoeopathic treatments which could be used for headaches, and only a visit to a homoeopath will help to find the right one for the individual concerned. Extreme care and expertise is required as the success of a homoeopathic remedy relies on an exact prescription being given. Various homoeopathic remedies are now available at health stores; however, I would recommend visiting a qualified homoeopath, especially if remedies already tried show no improvement in the condition being treated. Generally speaking, an improvement should be found after four or five doses, after which the remedy should be stopped. In acute conditions, it is normal for the dosage to be half hourly, decreasing to once every two or three hours as improvements are seen. Homoeopathic remedies should not be taken before or after a meal, with tea or coffee - the drinking of which should be discontinued whilst the treatment is in progress - or after brushing teeth. Remedies should be stored out of direct sunlight, away from strong smelling substances and aromatherapy remedies. Those interested in the science are encouraged to seek further reading on homoeopathy.

Making Your Own Cosmetics

Many people like to use flowers and natural substances in their skincare preparations. One of the benefits of using natural substances is that you can ensure, especially if you make the preparations yourself, that you are not using chemicals or substances which could cause allergy. Likewise, people who are against animal testing will have the added satisfaction of being sure that their products have not been tested on animals. However, it is necessary to realise that without preservatives home-made preparations will not have a long life.

For most of the preparations all you need is a heatproof bowl and a saucepan, together with normal kitchen utensils, storage jars and bottles. You may wish to use essential oils and I would strongly urge you to use a pure essential oil, not a fragrance oil or blend. If you are going to be storing your creams and lotions in a bottle or jar which has been used for other things, make sure that it has been properly cleaned and dried before use.

Cold Cream

It is best to use a blender if you have one. Failing that, a whisk can be used.

Ingredients:

Aloe vera gel (available from most health stores)
Corn or olive oil
White beeswax (available from chemist's or health stores)
Water-free lanolin
Rose or lavender water
Essential oil

Mix together a tablespoon of aloe vera gel and 150 ml of corn or olive oil. In the top of a double boiler, melt a tablespoon of white beeswax and 2 tablespoons of water-free lanolin. Slowly stir in the oil and aloe mix, remove from the heat and add 2 tablespoons of rose, lavender or other flower water, and 2 or 3 drops of essential oil. Stir until the mixture cools and thickens, before putting into jars.

A Moisturiser

Ingredients
gelatine
essential oil (rose works well)
glycerine

Dissolve a teaspoon of gelatine in 150 ml of hot water and mix in a teaspoon of essential oil and 3 tablespoons of glycerine. Alternatively, you may wish to mix equal portions of glycerine and rose water if you only wish to use the cream for hands. Reducing the amount of glycerine makes a less greasy cream, and you should experiment to obtain your preferred consistency.

A Toner

Ingredients
4 tablespoons of dried sage or 8 of fresh
(You can also use camomile for a less strong preparation)

150 ml vodka
Tincture of benzoin (available from chemists)

Put 4 tablespoons of dried sage into a clean jar and add the vodka. Make sure that you tighten the lid well, and leave to stand for a week. Then strain off and remove the sage, adding the same amount of herb as before, and leave for another week. Repeat the process once again. Strain the liquid into a bottle, using a fine sieve (coffee filter paper can be used if you don't have a sieve). Add 4 or 5 drops of benzoin tincture, screw on the lid and shake well. Adding a couple of tablespoons of witch hazel strengthens the mixture.

A Deodorant

Ingredients
gentian tincture

Taking a mixture of 10-12 drops of gentian tincture in 1 cup of water 3 times a day before meals will aid food absorption and will help with body odour, which stems from this.

A Face Pack

Ingredients
100 g camomile flowers
(Suitable for all skin types, even sensitive skin)
Strips of gauze

Put your flowers into a heatproof dish, pour over enough boiling water to form a mash, and leave for 10 minutes. During this time, moisturise your face. Spread the mash over strips of gauze and place on cheeks, nose, chin, throat and forehead. Leave this on your face until it cools, which will take around 20 minutes.

Should you wish to try a more adventurous face mask, you will need a dry base. Oatmeal and ground almonds are suitable for most skin types.

Ingredients
Oatmeal and ground almond mix
Egg yolk
Natural yogurt
Rose water

Open the pores of your face by standing over a bowl of steaming water for a few minutes or applying a warm, wet face cloth to your face for a couple of minutes. Combine 3 tablespoons of the oatmeal and ground almond mix with water to make a thick paste, and add the other ingredients. Spread the paste well over your face and neck, avoiding the lips and eyes. Leave on for 25 minutes, or until dry completely, then gently wash off with warm water. Ideally, face packs should be used on a weekly basis. Oat bran, oatmeal and ground almond will not cause a reaction on sensitive skins. For exceptionally sensitive skins use oat bran and boiling water, which has been mixed to form a stiff paste. Apply to the face, and wash off after 10 minutes with lukewarm water.

A word here on allergies - allergies can be passed on from parent to child and 10-12 drops of gentian root tincture, available commercially, taken 3 times daily before meals can reduce the likelihood of this happening if taken before conception and while nursing. This remedy is also said to be useful if taken by mothers nursing babies with eczema or other skin complaints.

A Cleanser

Ingredients
Beeswax

Liquid paraffin
Any essential oil, but lavender works very well
A double boiler

Using a grater or sharp kitchen knife, make 8 tablespoons of grated beeswax. Heat gently with 450 ml of liquid paraffin in the top of a double boiler until melted. Cool to 50°C while separately heating
300 ml of water to the same temperature. Slowly add the water to the wax and oil mixture, stirring continuously, then add a couple of drops of the essential oil. Leave to cool until it begins to solidify, then pour into storage jars.
Another simple cleanser can be made using borage or cucumber.
Make a pulp of the plant and apply to the face. Slices of cucumber placed around your eyes reduce puffiness and redness, and will cool the skin.
Skin blemishes and spots can be brought under control with a little undiluted lavender oil dabbed straight onto the spot. A mixture of lavender and tea tree oil works well on cold sores. Lavender oil is nontoxic and can be used undiluted on even the most sensitive of skins.

A Facial Herbal Steam treatment

Ingredients
2 tablespoons fresh herbal leaves or flowers
1.25 litres of water
Non-aluminium saucepan

Bring the herbs to the boil in the water, simmer and cover for 3 minutes. Pour the contents of the saucepan into a heatproof bowl and hold the face about 20 cm above the water, making sure the head and bowl are covered by a towel. Move the head from side to side, taking care to keep the eyes closed. Do this for 5-10 minutes, then rinse the face with warm water, pat with cold herb tea, and dry. It is best to leave the skin free from other cosmetics or extremes of temperature for at least an hour.

Herbs to consider for the steam treatment are:
- Normal to dry skin Chopped comfrey leaves or root with camomile flowers in equal quantities
- Sensitive skin Borage leaves and flowers or sorrel
- Difficult skin Equal quantities of chopped comfrey root, crumbled lavender flowers and chopped lemon grass

A Hair Tint

Ingredients

200 g of chosen herb (see below)

Make an infusion using 200 g of herb to 500 ml of water. Rinse hair regularly in this mixture. To achieve a good hair colour create a paste made from the herb and leave on the hair for around 30 minutes. As with any hair colorant, it will need to be reapplied when hair growth is apparent.

Henna paste (powdered henna, mixed with water) with camomile infusion or lemon juice - *brings out the auburn in hair*
Henna paste mixed with hot black coffee - *deepens hair colour*
Henna paste mixed with indigo from the root of the indigo plant at a ratio of 1:3 - *tints hair from dark brown to black*
Camomile paste with kaolin powder – *highlights mid-brown hair*
Marigold flower infusion or saffron roots or flowers – *gives reddish tint to white hair*
Walnut bark infusion - *darkens grey hair*
Rhubarb root infusion - *lightens any colour hair slightly*
Sage infusion - *gives brown tint to grey hair*
Sage infusion mixed with tea - *deepens the colour of brown hair*

If you have greasy hair and/or dandruff, you may wish to try an infusion of 60 g of camomile to 600 ml of water extracted for 15 minutes, as a rinse. Another solution might be to rub chickweed lotion into the scalp before bedtime and next morning wash the hair with a chickweed shampoo.

Stressed hair is easily restored to health by using a small amount of blended lavender and sweet almond oil over the scalp, through the hair to the roots, then combing to the ends. Wrap the hair in cling film and a warm towel, and leave for 20 minutes then shampoo away and dry.

A Bath Treatment

Ingredients
60 g herbs
Boiling water

You may use essential oils, herbs and herbal infusions as part of your bath routine, and you can experiment with different types of herb and different oils. Make the infusion for a bath using 60 g of herbs to 600 ml of boiling water, leave for 30 minutes, strain and add to the bath water. Alternatively, you may make a little herbal bag using muslin, and hang it over the tap so that the water runs onto it as you draw your bath. If using essential oils, a couple of drops is quite enough, and remember to relax in the water, whether you are using the herb infusion or the essential oil. A camomile infusion in a bath is especially good for those suffering from rashes, and is well worth trying with children.

A Skin Revitaliser with Fruit

Ingredients
Lots of strawberries

Fennel seed tea

You may wish to try this quick and easy fruit revitaliser after you have cleansed and/or steamed your face. Make a pulp of the strawberries, using enough to cover your face and neck, leaving the eyes, lips and nostrils clear. Place cotton wool pads which have been soaked in cold fennel seed tea on your eyes. Leave this on your face for 20 minutes. Rinse off with warm water and splash the face with cool water. Your face will feel totally refreshed. You may also try other fruits such as apricots, bananas or tomato pulp. You can mix these with an egg white and thicken with wheat flour – use two tablespoonfuls of pulp to one egg white.

Chapter 3 – Flowers and Meditation

It is quite easy to use flowers in meditation by using guided imagery or creative visualisation. Meditation and relaxation techniques are involved subjects, and it is important that the complete novice acquires as much information on the subject as possible, as it will not be possible in the space we have available to discuss all the intricacies of meditation.

For those who are a little unsure about meditation, please be assured that it is not connected with any religious philosophy but is something which will help us and our general wellbeing and something that we are all capable of achieving, irrespective of faith or religious belief. Learning to relax and to meditate is something which will benefit everyone. Meditation is not about learning chants, communing with 'higher forces', belonging to sects, groups or organisations, or opening the mind to potential evil influences. It is simply something which you can do in the privacy of your own home to help you personally to relax and enjoy life a little more by reducing the stresses and tensions, which are part and parcel of living at this time.

Learning to relax

Before embarking on a period of meditation, it is important that you learn how to breathe properly and how to relax by concentrating on your breathing patterns. Different people have different ways of initiating the relaxation process, and what follows are some suggestions of techniques which have worked for my colleagues and myself.

In order to relax properly we need to breathe in a slightly different way from the way we might normally breathe. Everyone breathes differently. Some people naturally take shallow breaths, some people breathe from their stomach area, whilst others breathe from their chests. People also breathe at different rates depending upon the circumstances. If scared, physically active or tense, the rate of our breathing will rise. The rate of breathing can also be affected by fitness levels. Some people, especially those who are overweight, will find that they might breathe faster than others. This is all part and parcel of being unique as an individual.

When we are talking here about relaxation, what is it we are talking about? Relaxation isn't about sitting in front of the television, reading a book, having a drink with family and friends or listening to music. Whilst we might feel that we are relaxed, all we are really achieving is a state of being more relaxed than we were previously. Total relaxation is what we are talking about when embarking on a period of meditation.

Science has shown that during total relaxation, our brain waves change. For example, when we are asleep we are in an alpha state for much of the time, changing to a delta state when we are in a deep sleep. What we are endeavouring to achieve by total relaxation is a controlled alpha state.

Before we start to relax, we need to make sure that we have given ourselves permission. Many of us live such a hectic life that in order to get into our day everything we wish to achieve we try to avoid anything that slows it down. Nothing wrong with that, but what we must also realise is that to operate effectively, we need to relax, otherwise we might suffer from burnout. Burnout comes in a variety of differing guises: some people might find themselves bothered by migraines, other people might find themselves permanently angry and wound up by things all the time. What is happening when we get these symptoms? More often than not, this is part and parcel of our body trying to tell us that we need to find time to relax. There is nothing wrong with programming into a schedule a little time for yourself. You aren't being selfish; you are just trying to help your body to operate a little more effectively. If you come to realise how important you are not only to yourself, but also to your family and your friends, you will realise that you owe it to yourself to be as effective and as healthy and well as you can. I would like you to try a little experiment to help distinguish your feelings of tension. I want you to imagine yourself in a frightening situation. Some of you might have a problem imagining anything at all, in which case, I would suggest that you watch a scary film for a while. Every now and again, check to see whether your breathing is the same as it was. Be aware of your body's reaction when you are scared. Do your shoulders come up, do you clench your fists, do you shout out loud, jump up, cover your eyes. Make a note of how you feel and how your breathing changes. What you should find is that you are tense. When you are tense your breathing becomes more shallow. You enter into what psychologists and students of human behaviour call the 'flight or fight' mode. You may want to jump up, leave the room, switch the television off or do something else because you feel tense.

Now let's try another little experiment. I want you to lie down somewhere warm and where you won't be disturbed. Some people feel that lying down makes a subconscious association with sleep, and we don't want anyone to drop off to sleep. If you find lying down problematic you may wish to try sitting on a chair. If you decide to sit on a chair, make sure it is comfortable, and do not cross your arms or legs, as not only will this hinder your circulation, but it can also prevent total relaxation.

Take the telephone off the hook, ensure that you won't be bothered by the demands of your family or pets, and that you have IS-20 minutes to carry out the experiment. For the first few times you may wish to tape the following passage and have it playing to you as you go through the experiment so that you can totally let go. Once you have done this a few times it will become easier and this won't be necessary. Don't rush this experiment!

Remain still for a while and try breathing in to a count of five, hold your breath for a seconds, and then breathe out for a count of five. Do this a few times. You may, if you are unaccustomed to such breathing techniques, feel a little light-headed, but as you are lying or sitting down don't worry about this too much. When you feel happy with the position you are in and feel that your rate of breathing has slowed down a little, try squeezing up your toes. Hold that squeeze for five seconds and then release it. Next, I want you to tense your calf muscles by keeping your feet and legs on the floor and pointing your toes upwards towards your face. Hold for five seconds and then release. I now want you to squeeze your knees together as hard as you can, hold for five seconds and then release. Now squeeze your buttock muscles together as hard as you can. Don't worry about what anybody might think if they saw you, just squeeze and hold it for five seconds then let it go. Next, I want you to imagine that you are going to have someone stand on your stomach. It will be really painful unless you tense your muscles so tightly that the person will be supported. Do that for five seconds and then release. Make a fist with your hands and squeeze tightly. Again, hold for five seconds and then release. Bring your shoulders up to your ears and squeeze as tightly as you can for five seconds and then let go. Clench your teeth together - some people call this setting your jaw. Again, keep this position for five seconds and then release. I want you to close your eyes tightly, as if you are trying to keep all the light out. Hold for five seconds and then release.

You have progressively tensed and relaxed most of the major muscles in your body. Remain lying down for the next few minutes and think about how much better it feels to have relaxed rather than tensed muscles. In time get up gently, making sure that you don't leap up, try to curl up like a bulb growing from the ground, and lift your head and neck last. By making sure that your head and neck come up last, you will prevent any light-headedness. The whole experience is about calm and peace, and you should make sure that you take your time, acclimatising yourself to the room again after your relaxation period before getting up and carrying on your day. You may wish to stretch or shrug your shoulders a little. Once we have mastered this sort of technique, we can progress as this is only the first stage in what we are setting out to achieve. When in this relaxed state, we can further our imagination, concentrate on things which we find pleasurable, places we have been or guided imageries, and we can relax a little more deeply.

Creative Visualisation

For the purposes of this exercise I want you to think in terms of flowers and about creative visualisation. This means thinking and concentrating on one thing within your mind and that alone. We all do it at times. Some people call it daydreaming, but when in a daydream we are often thinking about a series of things, people, places or events. For this experience, we are talking about focusing attention on one thing, and this is to be a flower. Most people, new to this practice, can find it difficult but after practice it becomes a lot easier.

The choice of flower is a personal one. You should try to choose a flower you like because we are aiming for a positive experience here - avoid anything associated with unfortunate events or people. I personally use a pink rose: roses to me are beautiful things, connected with love and warmth of feeling; the colour pink is associated with unconditional love and emotion; the two, in my mind, link well together. If you like a particular flower and are not bothered too much about the colour angle, don't worry. If, however, you wish to introduce some colour into your body for the wellbeing that this can bring, try to think of a flower and colour which are real, rather than something you know doesn't exist. The flower you choose can be a flower we have around us now, a seasonal flower, or it can be a flower that we only see at certain times of the year. It can also be a flower we've seen on travels abroad, on television, or a flower which has a significance for you from another sphere of your life.

Make sure that you are comfortable with the exercise we discussed in progressively tensing and relaxing your muscles. Make sure that the place you have chosen for your meditation is somewhere quiet with no distractions. Obviously, you can't control the outside and traffic noise cannot be stopped, but try to find a time of day when you will be relatively sure that you will not be distracted. Make sure that the period you choose for your meditation is one when you haven't previously felt rushed. It is useless to come in from a day at work feeling flustered and uptight, and then try to meditate. Unless you are very experienced you will find it virtually impossible to meditate unless you have a passive attitude. We need to get rid of the day, and for this reason many people choose to meditate in the morning before the 'cares of the day' get hold of them. People also feel that meditation sets them up for the day, but again I leave it up to you to decide for yourself. Find a time which suits you, and also make sure that it is a time which suits your family.

Getting Started on a Visualisation

At this stage, I hope that you have chosen your place, time and object. You can choose to think in terms of one flower or several. If you do choose several flowers, I would suggest that you think in terms of one type of flower rather than a mixed bunch, at least until you feel comfortable with visualisation techniques. Some people have difficulty in visualising something unless they have the opportunity of seeing it beforehand. If you feel that might apply to you, you may wish to have the chosen flower or a picture of it, in front of you. Look at it carefully and familiarise yourself with it before you start to relax. Start by going through the relaxation process we have developed. Once you feel comfortable with this process you can develop your own techniques - you need not stick with the guidelines suggested earlier.

Meditation with a Flower

Once relaxed, close your eyes and think about your chosen flower. If you have a problem with closing your eyes, do at least try to keep your focus away from anything which could distract you, such as a room in which the wallpaper is heavily patterned.

Really focus your mind on the colour of your flower. Imagine that the colour you have chosen is permeating your body so that you are totally enveloped by it. Try to imagine the smell, and breathe in deeply, breathing in the smell of the flower, its colour and its form. Examine the structure of the flower - its petals and its form. Think of the petals one by one, and look how they are held together at the central point. Look at how the colour of the petals alters in certain areas due to the type of flower itself, and how the light is falling on it. Look at how some of the petals may curve downwards whilst other newer petals may still be close to the centre. If you have chosen a bud as your flower, try to imagine that during the course of your meditation the bud opens and the flower comes into full bloom. Look at the stamen. Look at how the flower meets the stem. Look at the stem in its glory. If you have chosen a flower with thorns, look at these and see how they protect the stem. Look at the leaves, see them as individuals and see how they join onto the stem. Look at the colours of the leaves. See the whole flower, stem, petals and leaves as an entity and see yourself as one with this flower, part and parcel of a whole.

I would like you to stay with this meditation for at least 20 minutes, although this is a guideline, and not a hard and fast rule. I would strongly advise against having anything that will tell you when your 20 minutes is up. The ringing of a timer can cause problems by bringing you out of the meditation too quickly. Come out of the meditation in your own time.

When you come to the end of your meditation, make sure that you sit and breathe deeply for a while, acclimatising yourself to the room and your surroundings. It is not advisable to leap up and go and carry on with the day. Take time with the whole experience, including the period afterwards. You may wish, upon opening your eyes again, to have a bit of a stretch, wiggle your toes, clench and unclench your hands, move your shoulders about, or yawn. Do whatever you feel happy with and remember to take your time. This is time you have allowed for yourself. You should not feel guilty at the end for the time you have taken, so just let the whole experience unfold as it should.

You may wish to do this meditation daily. You may, on the other hand, feel that you only want to do this once a week or when you have the time or inclination - this is fine. Some would suggest that we should meditate every day at the same time in the same place. Although there may be bona fide benefits to doing this, it would be unwise to decide upon a schedule which you know you can't stick to, and which will lead to you giving up on meditation altogether. Be realistic in your goals and feel free to alter the goal posts if necessary. Many years ago I worked in an office and my colleagues and I decided to go to a relaxation class which was held on a Friday lunchtime. We decided that this would be more constructive than rushing round the shops or going to the pub. Although it was a very good class we found that we were unable to gear ourselves up again in the afternoon without getting dreadful headaches and feeling ill. This was because we didn't realise that our bodies would be so relaxed that we would find it virtually impossible to get going again. It wasn't a wasted experience as we have all carried on meditating, but at times which are more suitable.

Stick with meditation and don't be discouraged if you find it a little more difficult than you thought at the outset. Never compare yourself to others as this is not a competition. Remember that we are all different. If you persevere your visualisation techniques will improve and your health and wellbeing will improve.

Once you feel happy with the art of creative visualisation, you may wish to embark on other visualisations which involve more than one object. Visualisations can involve a mental journey as well as an object. We are now going to look at a sample visualisation using a journey. I would, however, advise readers who are new to meditation to stick with one flower until they feel happy moving on.

Meditation with a Journey

This meditation is about going to a place, and we will go beyond where we have been before. There are two ways of doing this: you may choose to return to a place where you have been before, or you may wish to go to somewhere where you have never been, but would like to visit. Some of us find that when we return to places where we have been, we think of people who are no longer part of our lives and this can cause us upset. As we wish to avoid this, you may wish to think of somewhere you have never been before. However, most of us will probably have been somewhere where we had a great time. It might have been a holiday or somewhere we lived before. It might have involved other people or conversely it might have been something you did alone. I want you to decide the place and the time yourself. For example, I had a particularly lovely holiday several years ago in Crete. I remember being on a motorcycle, coming down a long road from a series of hills and seeing the bay below and the sea shimmering in the distance. When I close my eyes even now, several years later, I can still picture that place and feel the sun and the wind on my face.

I want you to think for a while about which particular memory or event has had a happy impact on you. We will not be reliving this experience, so simply take a mental snapshot, excluding the whole day's events, conversations or people. Even if you were with other people, try and imagine yourself alone. If you have difficulty visualising a place, you may wish to look at some old photos and choose something from amongst them. You may wish to look at a holiday brochure as some people feel happier with something that they can't relate to themselves and some people seek to take themselves off somewhere that they know they are unlikely to ever visit, but would like to see. You may wish to try going somewhere you have only seen on a television holiday programme.

Go through the whole process of relaxation again. Make sure that you have chosen your time and that you will not be disturbed. Just breathe for a few seconds, take your time and close your eyes if you feel comfortable. See yourself as weightless. Become part of your chair or the ground on which you are lying. You have no form, no weight, and you can float. You are unable to move, because you feel so relaxed. After a while imagine yourself able to float off anywhere, in the past, present or future. You are weightless, lighter than air, and you can take yourself out of your present surroundings, up above the clouds and float off. You are warm. You are weightless. You can go anywhere, and do anything.

Take yourself off in that state to the place you have chosen to visit. I want you to stay in that cloud formation. You are above everything. You can look down at the place you have chosen to visit and see it in its beauty. Take your time to look at the scenery, look at the colours, hear the sounds and take it all in. Stay there for a while, looking down in that position. There is nobody else there in your scene - all you can see are the flowers, trees and views. This is the place you have always wanted to be. This is total paradise. You can see everything, and there is total peace and quiet around you. Take in the picture, and be a part of it. Look at the beauty of the colours, listen to the sounds. Feel happy. Be relaxed. When you feel comfortable, you may wish to take yourself down from the cloud structure and become a part of your scene. You may wish to relax there or you may wish to take a walk around and look at everything there is to see there. Take as long as you like doing that. Enjoy the experience. Be warm, happy and calm.

When you feel you wish to move on, tell yourself that it is time to leave, give yourself permission to leave and permission to return at a future time, and take yourself back into the weightless structure amongst the clouds. Look back down at your scene. Drink it all in, see all the things you have seen from the ground, and then move back to where you really are, and bring yourself back down into the room. Stay in the room, and take a few deep breaths, breathing in to a count of five and out to a count of five. Before opening your eyes, you may wish to have a stretch, a yawn, wiggle your toes and fingers and move your shoulders up and down. Make sure you take your time with this, and that you don't just leap up. When getting up, uncurl yourself and make sure that your head and neck come up last.

What we have achieved is to take you through guided imagery, using scenery and tranquillity. You should feel like you have had a mini holiday. The benefits are that it hasn't cost you anything and that you haven't been troubled by anything.

When I carry out this meditation, I always take myself off to a beach scene. I see the white sandy beach, palm trees and sunshine. I see a lovely blue sea and a cloudless sky, and I feel myself lying on the beach, or sometimes in a hammock strung up between two palm trees. I take it all in, listening to the gentle lapping of the waves on the shore, taking myself to a time when the sun is just going down - it is still lovely and warm, and the sky is changing colour to reds, yellows and golds. I have a tape which I sometimes use as background with the sound of ocean waves, and I use this actively to help with the meditation. Although other people might find this distracting, I find that it helps me, and helps me to hold on to the image I am creating. It lasts for about 20 minutes, which is as long as I take over the visit to my beach. There are several tapes which you can purchase with just sounds of nature on them. I have friends who use tapes of English country gardens, with bird song on, and they use these to create guided imageries of visits to various parts of England during various months of the year. Again, this is a personal thing, and you might find that having sound in the background is not right for you. Experiment and find what suits you.

I would suggest that, as you progress, you occasionally introduce a new journey into your meditation, and we will now give a few suggestions that you may wish to try when you feel happy to progress using seasonal thoughts.

Other Meditations

As you progress with meditation, you may wish to incorporate seasonal factors. If you are lucky, you may live near an area of natural beauty. I am fortunate in that I live on the outskirts of a wood which forms part of a National Forest. I can walk out of my door and within a minute I can be in woodland, where I can walk for hours without coming across anybody else, other than the occasional dog walker. I often think that those woods are the nearest thing to paradise I might ever get to see within England. There are squirrels in the wood, and occasionally you might see a fox. There is also the ruins of an old priory, and cattle now graze around that area at certain times of the year. There is a stream running through part of the wood, and it is lovely to stand on the little ornamental bridge which leads up to a more cultivated area, and watch how the water hits the rocks and stones and splashes up onto the bank before continuing on its journey. Closing your eyes and just listening to the sound of the water, with the birds making their cheery noises in the background is quite an experience. There are many different varieties of trees, some really old and splendid, whilst others are relatively young, and there is one tree in particular which I love to visit. It is an old oak tree, strong and tall, with branches which seem to spread out over a huge area, touching the ground in some parts and reaching out in other areas to just skim the branches of neighbouring trees. I call the tree Peter, much to the amusement of people I have taken walks with in that wood. I look on him as the foundation of the wood, in the same way as there are those who may think of Peter as the foundation of the Christian church. When I go to that area, I make a point of feeling the bark of the tree, looking at the marks on it, and thanking it for its presence and its beauty. There are also lots of shrubs and bushes. The woods change with the seasons, and the same area can look totally different in different seasons. In the summer months the rhododendron bushes are a delight to see, as the colour they bring to the area is magnificent. In the spring, the woods are full of bluebells, and in the autumn, the changes in the colours of the leaves makes a lovely sight. The wood also changes in winter. The snowfall and the ice make everything crisp, and walking in the woods you can hear the cracking of the twigs under your feet and feel the crisp air on your face. There are some snowdrops, the holly berries add colour, and the whole scene is like a painting. When it seems cold and dismal outside, it is nice to meditate on the woods, taking myself back to another season when I can look at the colours, at the flowers and trees, and relive the happiness of being in the woods at that particular time of year.

I am lucky that I have this on my doorstep. You might not be so fortunate, but I am sure there must be somewhere that you have been, which would create the same meditation for you.

Seasonal meditations can be great experiences. Make sure you think not only in terms of the place that you are visiting but that you also think in terms of the flora and fauna around you, the colours and the smells and the feeling of peace and tranquillity. I would advise against thinking about visiting an area when it is really cold, unless you have practised meditation for some time and feel comfortable with including heat variations into the theme without it physically affecting you.

During the course of this chapter, we have taken a brief look at meditation using flowers and surroundings. I would like to stress again that this is only an initial guide to meditation and the many varied types of meditation you might wish to employ for your benefit. Take time to enjoy the experience of meditation, and I would strongly urge those with an interest in meditation to undertake further reading.

Chapter 4 – Looking at Colour

During the course of this chapter, we will be taking a look at colour, delving into the world of Aura-Soma (oils which balance colour and the power of herbs), looking at giving colour to people in gifts of flowers and plants, as well as introducing colour into the home.

The Importance of Colour

Colour is all around us, but it is estimated that more than 2 million people in Britain alone are unable to identify colours properly. Colour vision is normal if you see white when three beams of light (red -long wave, green - middle wave and blue - shorter wave) are combined in equal proportions. When the three beams are blended in varying proportions other hues are produced. If, however, all the hues that are visible to you can be matched by mingling only two of these primary colours, and a third colour being added doesn't make a noticeable difference, then your colour vision is defective and you are termed dichromatic. Some people, like my father, see no colours at all and see things in various shades of grey, whilst others see only a few colours. Scientists tells us that of the 130 million light receptors in the retina, only 7 million give colour vision, and it is acknowledged that as we age, our sensitivity to colour alters, normally in relation to blue light.

Scientists have discovered that colours produce definite sensations, and blind people can be taught to 'see' colours by responding to each shade's vibratory rate. Experts suggest that we can all discover the ability to feel colour with practice. Red is sensed as a burning sensation, whilst orange is less hot and yellow feels almost tepid. Violet is said to be cold.

There are around 10 million tones, tints and shades, and we notice these sometimes at a subconscious level. At other times, striking colours grab Our attention and we immediately see the impact of the colour. You only have to take a drive or walk through the countryside to be bombarded with colour, especially during the spring and summer months. It is often the colour of the flowers that determines which insects are attracted to them, and it is also often the colours of nature which have the deepest effects on us. I especially like the carpet of indigo-blue that bluebells give, and also appreciate the lovely yellow tones which fields of rapeseed add to the landscape in the British Isles. Fields of corn or wheat, interspersed with red poppies are a wonderful sight to behold, and can often lift Our spirits as colour can affect us at a deeper level than the obvious visual impact it has. Many people who have studied the effect that colour has on our lives suggest that colour affects us on a deep, subconscious level.

Colour and Health

It has now become generally accepted by most people that colour can alter people's mental and physical health, and many people in business and commerce, as well as within the field of health and therapies use colour to bring out the best response in people. This all started at the very beginning of the 20th century, following on from work carried out by Rudolf Steiner. In the USA especially, some employers will go as far as engaging psychologists to carry out detailed assessment of job applicants by testing their colour preferences. It is now recognised that art therapy and the use of colours can help in establishing a balance between the physical and mental outlook of patients. It has been established that there is a definite link between certain colour foods and health benefits. For this reason, the Bristol Cancer Centre actively uses its knowledge of colour and health in the treatment and diet of cancer patients. It is now generally accepted that SAD (a seasonal deficiency illness, caused by lack of sunlight and colour) affects a great many people.

Many people suffer depression in months when it is colder and we have fewer colours around us from the world of nature, and most people will agree to feeling more optimistic and generally more buoyant when spring approaches. We can bring colour into our homes with plants and flowers and by actively seeking to change colour schemes to suit us more or create a feeling of harmony and balance.

Aura-Soma

Aura-Soma combines the power of herbs with the powers of aroma therapy and colour. It encompasses several products including rose waters, pomanders, quintessence and balance oils, but it is the balance oils which are our main concern here. Briefly, these oils seek to create a balance between colour and herbal oils. Known as balance bottles, it is felt that 'balance' can help us to create harmony. These balance oils, which can be used to work on the chakra systems of the body - the energy centres generally accepted to follow the line of the spine, or in other areas where imbalance is present - were developed by Vicky Wall, who had for some time been making herbal preparations, and was also a chiropodist and apothecary. All the oils contain essential oils and plant extracts, with an upper and lower fraction: the two balanced herb oils are placed within one bottle which, when shaken, will blend and then separate.
This is because the oily part of the plant is resting upon the watery part of the plant. Not only containing essential oils but also extracts from crystals and gems, these oils are important in terms of the energies of colour and light. They are designed to help replace the body's needs naturally from herbs, essential oils and using the power of colour, and they are recommended for use on any part of the body, especially for night application.

Colour is an important factor with the oils, and most people will be drawn to a particular bottle because the colours appeal at a subconscious level. These colour energies correspond, at a subconscious level, with the sort of person we are and with our needs. Most often, those interested in Aura-Soma will be offered a consultation, which will be based upon a selection of four balance bottles. Seeking to reveal difficulties of the past and underline strengths and gifts within the present, the colours will be explained and help given to enable the user to discover his or her full potential: the feeling is that we need to bring all the colours within ourselves to the surface so that we can begin to understand ourselves a little better.

Aura-Soma has 97 preparations which have been developed from an original S. There are some single colours and many dual-colour combinations. The original five colours of Aura-Soma were yellow over red (called sunset), yellow (sunlight), green over blue (heart), blue (peace) and violet over blue (Rescue Remedy).

To apply the 'balance', it is important that the two fractions within the bottle meet. This is done by shaking the bottle carefully, with the top open in a way which will be explained on purchase of the bottle. When shaken vigorously, a temporary emulsion will be formed and this should then be applied to the skin so that the oils and properties can be absorbed into the body.

It is generally accepted that colours give off different energies. These energies are known as colour rays. In order to benefit from rays, we need to know a little about each colour, how it can help us and how it can work against us. Armed with this information, we can take steps to bring that colour into our lives, either using Aura-Soma or by using flowers. We can also think about planning our gardens with that colour, or colours, in mind. Colour healing, also known as chromotherapy, is worthwhile considering, even if we are not seeking to use it on a daily basis. Broadly speaking, the warmer colours will help to vitalise and energise, whilst the cooler colours are calming and tranquil.

It is not possible to go through all the various combinations of Aura- Soma balance oils here, but we will take a look at the main prismatic colours - the seven colours of the rainbow - red, orange, yellow, green, blue, indigo and violet. These can be linked with various parts of the body and with the chakra centres. Those people who wish to understand all the colour combinations of the balance oils, should contact Aura-Soma direct. Their address is given at the back of this book.

Red

This has the longest wavelength and the fastest rate of vibration and the complementary colour for red is turquoise. There are many different shades of red, all of which fall into a similar category. Pink, however, made from mixing red and white belongs in a different category, and is the colour of unconditional love, unselfishness and spirituality.

Red will help with re-energising and is the basic energy colour for love, as well as lust. Although red at traffic signals indicates the need to stop, red as a colour has totally the opposite meaning as it is the colour of energy, of 'go'. Red is a very powerful colour, and it can be thought of as the colour of danger as it reacts with emotion, with passion and also with anger (seeing red). As such, it should be used with care, especially by those suffering from asthma, but it can help with impotence, chilblains, lack of warmth and energy, and with cramps as it helps to stimulate a sluggish circulation. It can also help us to earth ourselves, and is said to be particularly beneficial when used in sales offices as it will help with idea formulation.

Orange

This is the colour of the sun, and of light, heat and vitality, and the complementary colour for orange is blue. Orange is used in colour therapy fields for healing the respiratory system as it is a stimulant and reduces tiredness and depression. Working as a stimulant upon the adrenal area, it is said that orange can help lift the spirits, ease depression, release tension from muscles and help with hormone imbalance problems, and as such is often found in the offices of social workers and counsellors as it will help the clients. It is also useful in the treatment of digestive problems, and sportsmen and women may find this a particularly useful colour to aid with competitive events. Used by therapists in work with autistic children, too much exposure to orange can lead to selfish ambition and pride taking control. Said to be the colour which will aid relationships and help soothe relationship difficulties, those who are having a bad patch may be well advised to consider introducing some orange into their homes. It can also help in cases of shock, and can help those who are troubled to get themselves back together again.

Yellow

Stimulating, bright and cheerful, this is the colour of wisdom. It is also the colour of sulphur, which in alchemy symbolised creative energy. The complementary colour for yellow is violet. Yellow is often used by therapists to treat menstrual and menopausal problems, problems with digestion, blood pressure, the rate of breathing, the pancreas, liver and spleen. From a clothing angle, people are said to be either yellow or blue types, with yellow people looking good in yellow, gold and warm colours and not so good in purple or darker hues. Yellow helps with confidence, enhances concentration and wellbeing, and increases creativity and optimism. If you are feeling a little down, sitting near a vase of daffodils or other yellow flowers can often help. Yellow can help to lift our spirits, bring a little joy and happiness into our lives, and awaken us from a period of gloom and despondency. It helps with logical thought production, and is often termed the colour of decision making. It is also thought to help skin ailments, arthritis and weight fluctuation. Too much exposure to yellow will give rise to feelings of insecurity and loss of direction. Most of us will find yellow refreshing and will find ourselves naturally drawn to yellow, lemon, gold and sunlight colours in the summer months.

Green

Green is the colour of nature, the central colour in the colour spectrum and a great healer and promoter of restfulness. The complementary colour for green is magenta. Green acts as a stabiliser, a balancer between the positive and negative, it relieves tensions, helps with muscle building and is useful in cases of shock as it is a natural relaxant. Many hospitals use greens in their wards or waiting rooms as it is useful for those recovering from operations, and is a colour associated with healing. As most plants and flowers will have at least some green in their leaves and overall colour, it is not surprising that so many people bring plants and flowers into hospitals as gifts for patients. Certain theories suggest that green can help with the treatment of cancer patients. Green can be used by therapists in the treatment of headaches, colds and heart problems. It can help lower blood pressure and speed up the body's natural healing processes, and has been used to help in detoxification processes. Being the colour of many bank notes, green is sometimes associated with financial concerns and success. It is also said to be the colour of envy.

Blue

Blue is a spiritual colour, a good all-round healer, and is often called the colour of truth. The complementary colour is orange. Blue will help calm nerves, correct imbalances in the thyroid gland and lower blood pressure, as it is a natural tranquilliser. It will help to lift our spirits and give us faith and hope for the future, and will aid in the communication of true feelings. Most of us feel a little more optimistic when we see a blue sky than on grey days when there is no colour in the sky. Water, closely associated with the colour blue, will help to encourage peacefulness and tranquillity, and this is possibly one of the many reasons why beach holidays are so popular. Often found in solicitors' offices or in accountancy practices, blue in a room will give a feeling of confidence, sincerity and honesty. People are said to fall into the category of being a blue type or a yellow type. Those people who fall into the blue category will look good in blues and pinks but look bad in orange and brown. Blue is considered useful in the treatment of stress, tension and insomnia, and helps with infections, voice problems, rheumatism, fevers, burns and inflammations. Pale blue is said to be the colour of the conscience (as is turquoise) and helps to bring about a state of peace within. Royal blue is connected with more spiritual matters and things on a higher plane.

Indigo

Indigo is also known as midnight blue, and this powerful colour is normally associated with the unfolding of spirituality and wisdom. The complementary colour to indigo is gold. The colour of infinity and intuition, it is said that indigo can help with writing blocks, and is also a useful colour in meditation. It is used by colour therapists for healing emotional disorders, and is also used for sinus or respiratory difficulties, insomnia and headaches, diarrhoea and cystitis and can also help in cases of neuralgia.

Violet

This colour is associated with royalty, with mysticism and with religion. The complementary colour for violet is yellow. Violet links with peace, with the pioneering spirit and with serving others, especially if associated with matters of spirituality. Said to help us to learn to love ourselves as well as others, and to respect ourselves and boost our own self-esteem, violet will help balance the pituitary gland, help with nervousness and can be useful in meditation. Wagner and Leonardo da Vinci used violet in their surroundings for meditation. Too much purple or violet, especially in clothing, can help make those who are already a little sad even more depressed.

Colour in Our Food

We can take into our bodies the benefits of colour by the food we eat. At various cancer centres worldwide, an inclusion of red and orange foods into the diet of patients has given rise to exciting improvements in the health of those being treated. We should all, irrespective of whether we are ill or not, seek to introduce as many colours into our food as possible. We could start by thinking in terms of herbs and their flowers, but those people who are less adventurous can start by thinking of standard fruit and vegetables. Not only will the result be more colourful, but it can also be more healthy and add vital vitamins and minerals to our bodies. Obviously green foods are relatively easy to obtain, with peas, spinach, brocolli, cabbage, watercress and the like being obvious choices. There are many green fruits, from the common green apple or pear to something more exotic like the Kiwi fruit. These foods, as well as adding colour, also add vitamin C, vitamin E and in certain cases carotene. Brussel sprouts also contain B6, as does cabbage and spinach, and of course spinach is also a rich source of iron.

Cabbage is available in the red form, and tomatoes, beetroot and red peppers are also readily available. Many fruits are also red: from cherries and redcurrants through to plums and strawberries. Orange, in the form of carrots and swedes, is very beneficial to our bodies, and apricots, oranges and tangerines can be picked up easily at most supermarkets, irrespective of the season. Many of these foods, rich in vitamin C, are also a source of beta carotene, which is thought to help protect the body against illness. Yellow peppers, sweetcorn, lemons, grapefruit and melon all contain the yellow ray, whilst black grapes, blue plums, bilberries and blackberries will give us yet more variety of colours. Violet is available in purple grapes or plums, as well as aubergines and purple brocolli. Taking into account the benefits we can obtain by ingesting colour, and given the various illnesses which can be treated with colour, we would surely be doing ourselves a disservice by ignoring colour within our diets.

Colour in the Home

We have colour in our homes all the time and we also carry colour around with the clothes we wear. Often, we wear colour to make a statement. Business people will often be drawn to a particular colour, in order to get a message across subconsciously. We will also feel drawn to a colour when we need its help, and those people dealing with colour and image suggest that we will normally fall into the category of being either a spring, summer, autumn or winter person. This links us to the colours of nature, and has little to do with the time of year we were born. Spring types have peachy pink complexions, and normally blush easily. The eyes are normally blue or green, although occasionally hazel, and the hair will be golden blond, red or dark brown. These people look their best in off-white, beige, bright navy, turquoise, coral and red. Summer types have darkish hair and beige skin. The eyes are probably blue, green, hazel or grey, and they will be at their best in rose-beiges, lavender, greys, reds and blue tones. Autumn types are usually fair-skinned brunettes or redheads with freckles. Their eyes are usually brown or green and they look their best in beiges, golds, mustard, orange-reds and yellowy-greens. Winter types are olive skinned and include most dark-haired people. Winter types look best in clear colours like white, navy, black and primary colours.

Within the home, flowers and plants can reflect personalities. We think of the colour of artwork, fabrics and decoration, and in a later chapter, we will look at decoration in greater detail. Colour therapists recommend that blue, a colour we often find in bathrooms, probably because of the association of ideas with water, will help to soothe the eyes and mind, and so consequently a relaxing bath becomes just that. Pink is also often used in bathrooms, and will help with relaxation, even on those who are colour blind.

Chapter 5 – The Healing Garden

In this chapter, we are going to take a brief look at other ways in which you may wish to use flowers and plants in your life. We will be talking about making your own potpourri, drying flowers and herbs, making a herbal garden, using pots and containers to improve the overall appearance and beauty of the garden, and ways of making your garden something to enjoy. It is important to try to have a garden which holds interest and so retains its beauty and therapeutic value. The information given is only brief, and I would suggest that those interested seek further information. Remember gardens should be a paradise!

Making a Herbal Garden

I have a small herbal garden. I admit to not using it as much as I perhaps could, but it is an attractive and useful part of my garden, and provides fresh herbs to add to various meals and to use as infusions, compresses and inhalations. Herbs can look lovely just as plants and they can create a refreshing natural area in your garden or rockery. Adding a focal point, such as a seat or birdbath, can also help in adding interest to an area of herbs. If you intend to use your herbs, never take more than 20 % of the leaves from the plant, as you will be left with something in your garden which can be less than attractive. The following guidelines give some thoughts on what type of herbs you might wish to include in your herb garden and how you should go about it. You must first decide what herbs to use, and decide on the purpose of the garden. If you are looking for something which will create a lovely smell, you may think in terms of scented lavender or rosemary. If you want your herb garden primarily for culinary use, your selection will be very different. Those readers interested in a good selection of herbs are advised to consult their garden centre or undertake further reading.

Chives grow well in any garden and the flowers can be eaten. Sew the herb in March in rows about 6 inches apart. Many people will already have some parsley or mint in their gardens.
Parsley should be sewn in April for a summer crop and in July for winter and spring crops. Parsley will run to seed in its second year, and is best grown annually.
Mint will spread, so take care. Plant roots in March and cut all stalks down to the ground at the end of autumn. **Sage** should be planted in April and needs to be planted with room to spread - about one foot apart. Some gardeners suggest replacing sage every three years.
Thyme should also be sewn in April in a sheltered spot, and can also be planted in a rock garden. It is said to be good in treating depression and an infusion every now and then is a certain stress-buster,
Marjoram should be sewn in the spring in open, drained soil. Plant in May, having sewn under glass from March.
Fennel needs a sunny position and well-drained soil. It should be sewn in March with 2 feet between plants.
Tarragon makes a lovely plant for a garden as well as for a herb plot, as it has a lovely aromatic smell and greeny-white flowers in August. Planting in October or March will bring about a good plant, and remember that the leaves of this plant are suitable for freezing.
Rosemary needs a fairly large plot, as it can grow up to 6 feet in width as well as in height. Rosemary is another herb with a lovely fragrance. It needs to be planted in March or September in a sunny position, sheltered from strong winds.
Peppermint might be worthwhile considering for use in herbal teas and mint sauces, whilst **hyssop** leaves, picked before flowering, can be used in salads and sauces.
Basil works well with tomato in sauces, as those who like Italian food will well know.

Most herbs welcome a sunny aspect, and the soil should be moderately fertile and have good drainage. An ideal spot would be sunny and along the side of a wall or hedge. Herbs also flourish in pots. In order to create exactly the right soil, you might introduce a mulch of garden compost to the soil before you start, and you should make sure that you don't overfeed the herbs. Any space can be used, but make sure that you plant your groups of herbs around 45 cm apart to allow for growth. Also make sure that you plant smaller herbs near the front of your patch, so that they are not overshadowed by the larger herbs you might wish to grow. Consider making smaller groups of several types of herb. When buying your herbs, make sure you know what you are buying, and ask for help if necessary. Most garden centres are willing to give advice.

There is no reason why you should confine your herbs to one particular spot. You can plant herbs anywhere, and lemon balm, hyssop, parsley, marigolds, borage, feverfew, sage, chives, nasturtiums and others can add interest to a border in any part of the garden. Perennials such as lemon balm, feverfew, oregano, tarragon and sage are all suitable for borders. Scattering herbs between vegetables is another possibility. Dill can be sown between rows of carrots, lettuces or beans, and garlic always seems to thrive when grown next to strawberries. Other herbs can be scattered between rows of vegetables to create a little extra interest in the vegetable plot, and herbs worth considering for this could include camomile, coriander and aniseed. Lavender works well grown next to roses, whilst thyme and savory look good in rock gardens. You might also wish to change your lawn into a herbal lawn. Grassed areas were not originally a feature of country gardens and herbal lawns were very popular in days gone by. 'Lawns' can be grown from any plant, and a camomile or thyme lawn can look stunning. Traditionally camomile lawns were grown from the non-flowering variety called *Treneague,* which stays short, but as it can be expensive it is best grown from cuttings. Flowering camomile is cheaper and grows from seed. It creates a shaggy effect, and needs cutting with shears to remove flower heads for a shorter lawn. Thyme lawns are made from the species *Thymus Serphyllum,* but you can plant a mixture of other varieties to create a lovely carpet of colour. Herbal lawns are not hard-wearing, and if you walk across them regularly you might think about stepping stones. Wild gardens are another option. They are very popular at present, with many herbs and wild flowers planted together.

Lesser-known Herbs

Lesser-known herbs, such as ground elder, garlic mustard, tansy and horsetail can be unusual additions to your garden. Be careful with ground elder, as it spreads like wild fire through a wonderful root system. This means that the plant flourishes, even when you think you have pulled up all the visible roots. Buckwheat, once grown as a cereal, is also worthwhile considering, especially if you have poor sandy soil. The seeds contain a lot of protein and starch, and in days gone by was used to make flour for pancakes and bread. Agrimony is also worth considering. It was once considered an essential medicinal plant as the leaves were used to treat liver pains and gallbladder problems. *The* plant itself is wonderfully aromatic. Soapwort has pleasant light-pink flowers, which smell lovely in the summer months and are attractive to insects. *The* roots were used in ancient times for washing clothes, and it was thought the herb could cure coughs and colds. This plants grows to around 50 cm and grows well on most soils. *The* perennial Motherwort, also known as Lionheart, has lovely pink flowers throughout the summer, which attracts bees. *The* leaves were formerly used to treat heart problems, and can be used to make a calming herbal tea.

Those people who are suffering from depression and have already considered the use of St John's wort, might like to know that the variety best suited to treating such cases is *Hypericum perioratum,* which grows in dry soils and is normally found on heath land or on the edges of woods. It flowers around 24 June (St John's Day) and from this gets its name. This variety has five yellow oblong petals, and exudes a dark red juice when rubbed between the fingers. *The* leaves have tiny holes, which explains the name of this particular variety. To treat depression make an infusion from the petals and leaves, collected just before, or during, the flowering period. Finely chop the plant, and put a dessertspoonful in boiling water for ten minutes. Drink three cups of this infusion every day. Many press reports have suggested that this will help where other medication may fail, and it has no side effects, but I strongly suggest that people with depression talk to their doctor, especially if the condition seems long-lasting.

Herbs suitable for growing in pots include basil, bay, parsley, mint and thyme. Invasive herbs such as bergamot and oregano can be useful in pots, as this prevents them smothering other plants. Remember that your potted herbs are not indoor plants. If you treat them as though they are, you will end up with herbs that eventually turn yellow and die. They must have plenty of sun and air, and suitable places within a house are balconies, window ledges and patios. If you use pots, make sure that there is good drainage - make sure that the pot you use has holes in its base so that the water can escape. Terracotta pots are not really suitable containers, as they tend to dry out quickly on hot days. Hanging baskets can be ideal to use for herbs, but again you must make sure that there is plenty of water for them. When using a pot use a good rich compost, and add a handful each of grit and course sand for drainage. Half fill the pot with compost, then start to plant from the centre outwards.

A visit to the garden centre will help you make up your own mind on which herbs to consider, as well as being the place where you can ask for specific advice on herbs, their care and type of soils favoured.

Make sure that you remove old growth from your herbs regularly, as new growth is essential, and it makes for a better-looking plant overall.

Some people like to have a theme running through their garden. One idea is to make a planetary herbal garden. The following list of herbs show their traditional planetary links. Should you wish to organise the whole of your garden around a planetary theme, there are also details on trees and fruits which correspond traditionally to the planets.

Jupiter Sage, agrimony, balm, borage, hyssop, mint, dock, chicory, marjoram and chervil are often associated with Jupiter. Perennials such as oak, ash, fir, date, lime and fig also connect with Jupiter.

Mars Mars related herbs include sweet basil, tarragon, hops, blue flags, mustard, chives, soapwort, wormwood, garlic, yellow daffodils, gentian, ginger, marjoram, horseradish, pulsatilla and valerian. Peppers and onions also connect to Mars, as do nettles, box, broom, hawthorn, thistles and the pine tree.

Mercury Fennel, valerian, summer savory, mulberry, balsam, marjoram, oregano, caraway, southern wood, calamint, lavender, horehound, dill, red clover, vervain, comfrey, meadowsweet, tansy and parsley are often linked to Mercury. Trees which connect to Mercury include hazel, mulberry, myrtle and pomegranate.

Moon Hyssop, mistletoe, rosemary, lemon balm, saxifrage, clary, honeysuckle, chives, comfrey and witch hazel connect with the moon. Lettuce and cucumber also connect with the moon because of their high water content, as do watercress, water caltrops and lotus. Trees which connect with the moon include olive, palm, willow, privet and maple.

Neptune Meadowsweet, woodruff, burn et, lungwort, verbain, camomile, harts-tongue, liver wort, saxifrage and peppermint have all enjoyed links with Neptune.

Saturn Comfrey, quince, Solomon's seal (used to take the colour out of bruises), viola tricolour, mullein, henbane, ivy, monkshood, nightshade, *helleborus niger* (Christmas rose), elder, yew, yucca, beech, cypress, poplar, sloe, service tree, tamarisk, buckthorn, eucalyptus, holly and horse chestnut have all been linked with Saturn.

Sun Marigold, bay tree, borage, rosemary, angelica, rue, sorrel, fennel, St John's Wort, camomile, vine, ash trees, bay, juniper and walnut connect with the sun. Other herbs or spices, which connect with 'fire' are cinnamon, clove and patchouli. Citrus fruits such as oranges relate to the sun, and in warmer climes these might be something to consider.

Uranus Tansy, valerian, fumitory and horehound are connected with Uranus.

Venus Sage, clover, sorrel, yarrow, thyme, lovage, burdock, celandine, daffodils (yellow daffodils belong to Mars), peppermint, heather, dandelion, primrose, cowslip, pennyroyal and golden samphire. Apples, plums, figs, strawberries, alder, almond, apricot, blackberry, cherry, gooseberry, peach, pear, poplar, raspberry and sycamore also connect to Venus. Laurel, birch and rowan trees are also linked to Venus.
If you are interested in the Bible, and wish to plant a garden of Bible herbs, you might wish to consider sage, mint, dill, marjoram, wormwood, fennel, coriander and parsley.

Drying and Storing Herbs

If you want to dry herbs, you are well advised to do this on a dry day, and as early as possible in the morning so that any dew which may have gathered on them has evaporated and before any further heat from the sun dries the leaves. Choose only herbs which are at their peak, and remember that herbs can also be used when in flower as part of a dried flower arrangement. Feverfew, oregano, yarrow and mint work well in a bunch together, and make a lovely dried arrangement. Do not wash the herbs you intend to dry unless you might have used an insecticide on them, in which case the minimum of water should be used.

There are several ways of drying herbs. One of the most common methods is to take a bundle of herbs together, tie them with string, and hang them upside down in an airy but dark and preferably dust free place. I once tried drying herbs in the kitchen but found it too steamy. You may wish to put a paper bag around them, punched with holes, as this will protect the herbs from insects and dust. I find that this helps because any leaves which fall from the stem as the herb dries are not then lost, but can be collected in the bottom of the bag.

You can also dry your herbs easily in a microwave. Simply lay the herbs on some absorbent paper, and microwave them for around 30 seconds. Have a look at the herbs, and repeat this process until you can see that the herbs are drying out and crisping. Different powered microwaves lead to different timings here and some herbs take less time to dry than others. Consequently, I suggest looking at the herbs every 30 seconds, and when you see that the herb is becoming crisp, just microwave once more for 15 seconds.

Another way of drying herbs, is to put them on mesh trays in a warm place, out of direct sunlight, where the air circulates. Don't put your herbs in direct sunlight, as this will destroy the natural oils within the leaves. You can also use newspaper for drying your herbs. Drying time will depend upon the herb you use and the humidity. To store your herbs strip away the leaves by hand, and place them in dark glass containers. Make sure that they are clearly labelled, and always store them out of direct sunlight. If you wish to store fresh herbs, you can chop these and put them in plastic containers - they will keep in the fridge for about a week. Fresh herbs can also be frozen for up to three weeks - wash them, chop them finely and freeze them in ice cube trays in a drop of water. When you need to use them, just take out a herbal ice cube!

Drying Flowers and Making Potpourri

Many supermarkets and shops now sell dried flowers. Often you will find that buying dried flowers can work out rather expensive. Why not dry your own flowers, as there is nearly always somewhere in the home where a dried flower arrangement can go. Dried flower arrangements can make wonderful features, can be full of colour, and can contain many different types of flowers. It isn't very hard to make an attractive dried flower arrangement simply using foam and a small basket; or by placing dried flowers in a vase.

There are many different ways of drying flowers, flattening them out and leaving them there. Pressing flowers, which most people will have done at some time in their lives, can be quite a good way of keeping flowers, not only for sentimental reasons, but also for use in pictures and making personal cards. Many people will dry their flowers by hanging them upside down, as we have described with the herbs. Pick the flowers just before they turn into full blooms, and hang them upside down in small bunches in a dark dry cupboard, attic or garage. You must make sure that there is plenty of air circulation. The dryness of the environment will absorb any moisture quickly, and the darkness will help prevent the colours from fading. Leave your flowers hanging up until they are needed. You will be able to tell easily when they are dry enough to be used in decoration.

Another means of drying flowers, especially for the more open flowers like daffodils, pansies or Canterbury bells, is to bury them in borax. You will need a deep box, the bottom of which should be covered in powdered borax. Take all the leaves from the flowers and shorten the stems, then stand them on the borax and continue to put more powder around the flowers until they are covered over completely. Smooth out the petals as you cover them, so that they stay the same shape, and leave them in this powder for around three weeks. Then pour off the powder, and remove any excess with a soft brush. Be careful here as the petals will be brittle, and we don't want them to break off.

The final suggestion on how to dry the leaves is by using glycerine and water. This is a particularly effective way to deal with ivy, beech and laurel. Wash the leaves, remove dust and any broken or split pieces, and find a suitable jar or container. You will need one part glycerine to two parts water, which needs to reach about 10 cm up the stem. Keep the leaves in this mixture for around two or three weeks in a place where the air can circulate.

You can use dried flowers, not only in arrangements but also in potpourri which you can easily make at home. Potpourri can help with healing from a fragrance angle, and making it can be a therapeutic experience in itself. I usually use rose petals, and I use quite an old method. Mix 4 oz of kitchen salt with 4 lbs of fresh rose petals. Make sure the petals are not past their best. Leave for four or five days, then stir in a mixture made with 2 oz each of brown sugar, powdered orris, allspice, cloves, salt, bay and rosemary leaves. You can also use other sweet-scented flowers if you have these available. Stir the mixture well, add a handful of lavender and one dessertspoonful of verbena or other flower essence, and stir again. Cover the bowl, and the following day add 2-3 oz of brandy and stir again. Cover, leave until the next day and the potpourri should be ready. My 'recipe' suggests that to keep the potpourri fresh, you add brandy every now and again. You can also add fragrance oils to your potpourri or hide any small empty fragrance phials within the mixture.

Another fairly old-fashioned method of making potpourri, which has been used successfully in my family for many years, uses geranium blossoms, lavender, laurel leaves, wallflowers, acacia blossoms and delphinium petals, along with shavings of orange and lemon peel, and mint leaves. Keep this mixture in the airing cupboard on a shelf until the blooms are crisp, then mix together equal portions of powdered cinnamon, ground cloves, allspice, mace, kitchen salt and sea salt. Powder the flower petals together in your hands and stir, then pour a layer in the bottom of a large screw top jar. Add a layer of mixed salt and spices, and more petals, and continue with these layers until you have used up your mixture. A handful of this potpourri mix can be put into any small bowl, whilst the remainder can be kept in the jar for future use.

Scented Pillows

My grandmother used to make scented pillows, which she used to help pep up those suffering from illness. Crumble dried rose petals and mix with ordinary cloves, and crush with a heavy weight. Add a handful of dried mint, rubbed to a powder between the hands, together with some sweet briar leaves, dried lavender, geranium leaves, lemon verbena and any other sweet smelling petals. Add a little powdered cinnamon, orris, dried grated orange peel and any dried herbs, and stir. Empty into a small cushion cover so that it is stuffed tightly. If you need extra bulk, you can add chaff, fine bran or hay. Remember to sew up the ends of the cushion or pillow to seal it off. Sweet woodruff, a creeping woodland herb also makes good herb pillows, and is a useful ingredient of potpourri, smelling of new mown hay when dried.
You can also make a scented pillow for travel motion sickness, especially useful for children. Fill a small cushion with 50 g peppermint leaves, 50 g lemon verbena, 50 g lavender, 15 g mint scented pelargonium or mint leaves, 1 tablespoon crushed lemon zest, 1 teaspoon crushed nutmeg and 5-6 drops peppermint oil. Rest the head on the cushion during any journey.

Plants for Your Garden

If you are planning to change your garden, and wish to incorporate new ideas on aromatic plants, herbs or colours, you may be wondering what varieties of plants to use. What follows are just some brief guidelines on flowers and plants to use for the aromatic effect, plants to use for cut flowers, and what plants to consider if you are just interested in varying the foliage, colour or impact.

Plants with aromatic foliage Balm, eucalyptus, geranium, hyssop, laurel, lavender, marjoram, oregano, poplar, rosemary, sage, thyme.

Climbing plants with aromatic foliage Clematis, honeysuckle, climbing rose.

Plants with fragrant flowers Freesia, heliotrope, hyacinth, iris, jasmine, lavender, magnolia, narcissus, pansy, primula, rose, verbena.

Plants for cut flowers Anemone, aster, calendula, chrysanthemum, daffodil, dahlia, delphinium, gladioli, iris, lily, lupin, narcissus, phlox, tulip, verbena.

Plants with coloured foliage
Autumn colour - erica, larix, poplar, rhus. Grey or silver leaved - Artemisia, cypress, eucalyptus, saxifrage. Yellow or gold - juniper, thyme.

If you are looking for a pleasant scent, you can also consider using bark chippings in your garden. Blending in well in rockery areas, borders and around conifer trees or shrubs, the wood chippings give off a very pleasant woody smell, and they also make it harder for weeds to take over the garden. You could also consider making a pathway using bark chippings, but make sure that you have some grit underneath, and also think about inserting small wooden edgings to reinforce the boundary - garden centres can help you here. Planning a garden is a big thing and must be properly thought through. Garden design is a skilled job, and it is well worth seeking professional advice before making any firm decisions. You need to have a garden with which you feel comfortable, but you also have to take into account its care and usage. If you have little time to spare on a garden, you need to take this into account when in the planning stage, as it is pointless planning a garden to find that it takes too much of your time in maintenance and care. Consult a specialist, or at least visit a garden centre for advice before proceeding.

Eating Your Flowers

You may already use herbs and spices in your cooking, and include fresh herbs in salad preparations, but what about plants and flowers? I often eat nasturtium plants with salads, although some people think it strange. However, eating flowers is nothing new, but make sure that you are using plants and blooms which have not been sprayed with chemicals. The Romans ate lavender, Elizabeth I of England regularly drank lavender tea, and lavender biscuits are still occasionally found being baked in country kitchens. Lavender can also be used in sauces with fish and poultry, and green lavender can be used in stuffing mixes. If you wish to try this, mix a tablespoon of lavender leaves with a teaspoon of lavender flowers (either purple or green) removed from the head, and mix with butter, a little onion, egg and lemon rind. You can also use some lavender flowers (again removed from the head) in olive oil to add a little extra something when frying foods or making salad oil.

A flower petal salad can liven up a table - try using the flowers from chives, nasturtium, marjoram, marigold and borage, along with salad rocket, burnet leaves and gingermint leaves. Flower petals such as salad rocket flowers and marigolds can also be used. Lemon balm leaves, picked before the plant flowers, make an excellent accompaniment to salads, and can also be used in sauces and herbal teas. Salad rocket flowers can also be added to potato salads to make a difference. Heartsease (a violet pansy-type of flower) can be made into a tisane or again used in salads, and is especially useful in a garden because it self-seeds. Adding a few of the little blue borage flowers or pansies to the water in ice cube trays makes for an interesting finish to add to drinks, and borage is especially nice in elderflower tea. Borage flowers can also be used as a salad garnish, whilst the young leaves of borage taste similar to cucumber, and can be used to flavour drinks.

Oregano can be used to great extent by pizza-loving families – pick the leaves before the plant flowers and use them as a topping. They also make a lovely herbal tea. Pinks and rose flowers can be used to make jams, but be sure to remove the white heel from the bloom first. To make a rose petal jam, add 2 tablespoons each of orange and lemon juice to 150 ml of water and boil, together with 500 g of white sugar to make a syrup. Finely chop the rose petals, which should have already been gently washed and dried, and add to the mixture. Simmer for around half an hour, stirring continuously. Put into sterilised jars and seal as normal. Rose petals can also be crystallised to make a cake decoration, as can lavender flowers, by dipping them in egg white, then caster sugar and drying in a warm place. You might also wish to consider adding lavender flower heads to vinegar or oil to add a little extra flavouring. If using the petals of pinks try around 2 tablespoons in a little crème fraiche, and mix this with a fruit salad, using whole pinks for a little decoration.

Thinking of Seasonal Garden Colours

You may wish to organise your garden around seasonal plants and colours, so as to create a changing theme as the year progresses. It is necessary to plan this beforehand, making sure that the plants have their moment of glory without there being a patch where too many blooms are visible, or conversely without there being a time when there are no blooms visible at all. Remember, spring is the start of the gardening year, not January. Early *Galanthus, Eranthis* and narcissus bulbs can be a promise for the future, whilst herbaceous plants such as *Brunnera, Bergenia* and *Hellebore* can accompany early flowering daphnes, witch hazels and camellias. The plant commonly known as 'Edith Brogue' will continue to flower after the first part of spring, and it is important to make sure there is some continuity within the garden. Tulips, narcissus and flowering trees such as cherry, *Malus* and *Sorbus* are also worthwhile considering. If you are aiming for a huge area of colour in the summer months, why not plant some permanent shrubs such as shrub roses, rhododendrons (which like acid soil) and *Rosa* 'Chinatown', which grows to 3 metres in height. These shrubs work well with a perennial scheme, as do lilacs, peonies, laburnums and philadelphus. If looking for smaller plants and shrubs to place in front of the larger plants and shrubs, choose *Crocosmia lucifer* or *Lobelia cardinalis,* which grow to 90 cm, or *Achillea filipendulina* 'Gold Plate' which grows to 1.2 metres. Planting herbaceous perennials sets any garden area off, but remember that it will take around three years for the full effect to be achieved as it takes the plants this long to grow to their full height and spread. In the meantime, annuals and perennials can provide instant colour. Dianthus, lupins and poppies will keep the garden in bloom. There is also a flowering clematis for every season. Red flowers offer a touch of brightness for the summer. Red petunias are brilliant for filling in spaces. *Antirrhinum, Pelargonium, Lobelia* and *Pentstemon* are perfect for making a statement. Include some greenery to break up the banks of colour. Add depth and height with taller plants such as cannas, which have bronzed leaves on tall stems of red flowers. Dahlias are worth planting for a hot summer look. You can break up the redness of the garden area by introducing some purples and blues. Blue delphiniums and purple salvias work well together, and the foxtail lily will also add height to the garden. Roses are wonderful in a summer garden. If you plant smaller flowers such as irises or lavenders around them, they will truly make a statement. Later in the summer, fuchsias, hibiscus and hydrangeas make beautiful sights. Phlox, delphiniums, gentians, cyclamens, lilies and salvias can all bring texture and colour to the autumn garden. For later on in the year, consider asters and dahlias.

Creating Single Colour Schemes

If you prefer having one predominant colour within your garden, you may do a lot worse than choose white. White gardens have been popular since the famous white garden at Sissinghurst Castle in Kent was completed. White flowers amongst fresh green foliage creates a peaceful effect. There are white forms of tulip, iris, lily, peony, lychnis, phlox, *Zantedeschia, Leucanthemum,* poppy and veronica, which look wonderful en masse. Silver and spring-green leaves and white marked leaves make a stunning effect, especially if you remember to give equal space within the garden to the foliage. Consider the shape of the leaves, and include plants with spiny, feathery and frilled leaves. Worthwhile considering, in addition to those grey-leaved plants mentioned above, are Scotch thistle, *Artemisia* 'Powis Castle' and *Alchemilla mollis.* Early flowering white winter pansies and variegated honesty, white daisies and white tulips are a must for a spring show, and a few little forget-me-nets will add a little extra. White petunias and a splash of blue with *Onopordum acanthium* and *Hosta sieboldiana* will enhance the effect in the summer months. A white garden should also have a dash of powder blue in it, with a few geraniums or lavenders, as this will show the white flowers off to their best advantage.

Small Garden Ideas

If you have only a small area with which to work, all is not lost. Many people in urban areas have just a small patio area, which does not readily lend itself to becoming a garden for therapeutic help. If you think about introducing a variety of pots to the area, containing pentunias, bright ranunculus, marguerites, geraniums and Busy Lizzies or other such cheery flowers, you can easily transform what was a barren area into something far more pleasing to the eye and beneficial all round. Many garden centres will be able to supply patio roses, which flower for months, and can bring a burst of colour into an otherwise unattractive area. You can make a statement with even a single pot containing a mixture of flowers and evergreens, so that you will have a focal point all year round, not just in the summer months. Do not fill all of your containers with bright flowers – remember some greenery. This applies especially if you are grouping flowers together, and/or using containers of differing heights. If you use evergreens as part of your display, either within the same container or in a neighbouring container, the flowering plants will have more impact. Think about planting taller evergreen plants too. Conifers and climbers like ivies and vines work well, as do ferns on a slightly lower level.

You could also try placing pots filled with heavily-scented plants in an area where you might relax in the summer months, or conversely place such plants underneath your windows or next to doors leading into the garden, so that you get the full benefit when you open your door or windows. *Nicotiana* (the tobacco plant), or night-scented stock, honeysuckles, jasmine or roses around a doorway can add a great deal to the ambience of a room.

All container plants need watering daily, preferably in the early morning or late evening - but never in the heat of the day. If a plant is in direct sunlight during the height of summer, it may need watering twice a day. Also remember to feed your potted plants with a good commercial plant food regularly. Containers must have good drainage holes, which ideally should be covered with broken pottery or stones, a good layer of gravel and then fill with fresh potting compost. In my garden I have some old chimney pots, rescued from a house which was being demolished, and these make excellent containers for plants. In very large containers, such as barrels, half fill with garden soil, but the remainder must be filled with proper potting compost, and remember that once you have a large pot in position it will probably have to stay there, as it will be too difficult to move, so make sure the position is correct before planting them up. When using a patterned container, don't fill it with so many trailing plants that the container itself becomes lost. You can also use last year's growing bag in which you grew your tomato crop as a container. Planting some geraniums or petunias with ivy around the edges in such a container will easily disguise its origin.

To make the best of window boxes, choose a box which is the same width as the window, and plant up to suit the height of it as well. If you are thinking of creating a window box which will last all year round, ivy is a good choice with seasonal plants filling the spaces in between. Hanging baskets are also worth a thought, irrespective of whether you have a large garden area or no garden area at all.
Trailing plants such as ivies are good for hanging baskets, as are fuchsias and geraniums. You can also try nasturtiums which can be used in salads as well as being decorative.

Chapter 6 – Plants and Flowers for Decoration

Buying House Plants

I must admit that I am not particularly successful with pot plants. Those that last more than a month are likely to live forever. More often than not I am not successful in keeping them that long. I have, however, managed to keep a rubber plant for several years, and I have watched with fascination as many new leaves have come to life. Likewise, I am normally successful in keeping cactus plants - probably because I tend to forget to water plants. I also have two Clivia plants, which I have managed to keep for several years, and which produce lovely orange flowers if you allow the plant to rest - simply reduce watering and do not feed during the winter months. You may know many people like me, who whilst they appreciate flowers, cannot keep plants.

There is a theory that we give out vibrations which our plants pick up, and so consequently, if we are feeling negative about a plant, it will sense this and will perhaps suffer as a result. Plants watered by people suffering from depression, for example, have been shown to not thrive nearly as well as when they are looked after by someone in good health. Likewise, studies have suggested that if a batch of seeds are stared at in an aggressive way over a long period, they will suffer from inhibited growth as a result, whilst others will develop normally.

Talking to Plants

Many people talk to their plants. I do from time to time, and don't mind admitting it. It is said that talking to your plants and speaking kindly to them will be rewarded by a healthy plant. It could have something to do with faith, or perhaps it could simply be that we are giving our plants the carbon dioxide they need when we talk to them. Music is also said to help plants grow, especially gentle classics. Heavy metal music is said to make plants wilt! Many will scoff at this, but research indicates that plants are susceptible to communication and sound.

At Findhorn in northern Scotland, a community was set up in 1962 where giant cabbages, herbs and fruit grow even in freezing conditions. The soil is poor and sandy and the climate very harsh, but all the rules of nature have been broken by plants being grown and kept which most scientists said stood no chance at all of flourishing. Visitors to the gardens suggest that the spirituality of the community has a bearing on the plants and flowers, and as many as 50 different types of herb are grown there on a regular basis.

Colour in Plants

If you wish to introduce colour into your home in the form of a plant, the following are some which I would recommend, because they are colourful and not too hard to look after.

The winter-flowering begonia (also known as 'Glorie de Lorraine') has a profusion of lovely pale pink flowers which do not tend to drop quickly. The plant likes light but not strong sunlight and should be watered with lukewarm water, kept in a normally heated room, and fed weekly. Its cousin, the summer-flowering begonia can actually flower throughout the year, it has either red, pink or white flowers, and should be watered freely. It can be planted in tubs in the garden during the summer months.

Pelargoniums also have lovely flowers, in colours ranging from red and pink through to purple and blue. They are relatively easy to care for and can transfer outside into tubs in the summer months. They also keep well in conservatories and kitchens during the summer, but you must remember to water them well.

The cyclamen is normally found in the shops from September onwards, and needs a slightly heated room. It needs tepid water and does not particularly like being stood in a saucer of water because it tends to become cold. Cyclamens like sunshine, and again is one of those plants which needs a little plant food from time to time.

The crab cactus, which flowers in the winter, is another easy-care plant, and is best left to its own devices from mid-October throughout the winter. A little watering once in a while is quite adequate, and it will produce lovely pink flowers. African violets are another plant which normally flower well and can, if looked after properly, flower throughout the year. Flowers can be blue, purple, white, red or pink, depending on the variety. African violets should be kept in a dish as the soil needs to be kept damp with lukewarm water, and it also likes a humid environment. The faithful Busy Lizzie, also known as *Impatiens*, keeps well in most homes, although I must admit that mine have tended to go a bit 'leggy'. Flowering from spring to autumn, the plant needs to be kept in a saucer filled with water which is refilled daily, but any water left in the saucer at night should be removed. It likes a sunny spot, and can add a lot of colour to a room with its pink or orange flowers.

If you like to watch bulbs develop, the hyacinth is for you. Easy to grow, they can flower around Christmas time. Varieties of blue, pink, yellow, red and white are available, and when in full flower these are truly lovely plants.

Looking After Cut Flowers

As a general rule, in order to benefit from flowers and keep them longer in your home, you should pick them in the early morning or evening, when the sap is at its lowest. I always think that early evening is better. If you pick flowers in the heat of the day, they are more likely to wilt. Pick flowers relatively quickly, and get them into your home. Pick flowers which are just coming into bloom, rather than flowers in full bloom, as they will last longer. Give your flowers a long drink before you arrange them, irrespective of whether you have picked them or have bought them from a shop. Ideally, you should do this overnight.

Shop-bought flowers may have been conditioned before they are sold, but it is still a good idea to cut the stems under water. Using a sharp knife, cut flower stems at a sharp angle, so that the maximum area of the cut end is exposed to the water. Stand the flowers in a bucket filled with warm water and leave them overnight, or at least several hours. If the stems are a little bent and you wish to straighten them, wrap the flowers tightly in newspaper before putting them into the water. This is a very good tip for tulips.

If you are arranging gladioli, you should remove the topmost bud of the flowers to make sure that the remainder of the flowers will open. Flowers with semi-wooden ends, such as chrysanthemums, stocks and marigolds should have their stem ends scraped, which removes the outer substance and avoids slime forming. If using flowers which are laden with pollen, such as certain lilies, to avoid staining you can carefully remove the stamen if you feel that the pollen is likely to fall onto furniture.

If you are using poppies, a good tip is to make sure that the ends of the stems are singed over a flame. This is because they emit a milky sap which can cause problems with water intake. Poppies will also last longer if you plunge the stems into boiling water for a few minutes.

Drooping flowers can often be revived by placing them in shallow hot water for about half an hour, but you must make sure that the steam from the water does not interfere with the petals. A good way of protecting the petals from the steam is by wrapping them in paper. Take the flowers out when the water has cooled.

If you are arranging violets, remember that they absorb moisture through their petals when cut, so they need not reach water in any arrangement. If they wilt, you can revive them by submersion in water.

Always remove the lower leaves from flowers before putting them into the water. Leaves below the water line will rot and pollute the water, and will create cloudy water with an unpleasant smell and appearance. Roses should have their thorns removed with scissors, as well as the extra leaves and any little branches.

If you are using a lot of foliage, make sure that this is immersed completely in water for a few hours, as it will help it to last. The only exception to this is if you are dealing with silver-grey leaves.

Prolonging the Life of an Arrangement

You may be lucky and receive flowers as a gift. The arrangement should last for at least a week if kept in damp foam, or water. Most ready bought arrangements will have been conditioned, but to help them last a little bit longer, you must remember to use warm water, and ensure that all the leaves stay clear of the waterline. If you haven't been supplied with flower food, add a couple of drops of bleach and a teaspoon of sugar to the water to help prolong the life of flowers. Cut off around 2.5 cm of the stem and place in water for a good drink before making them part of any decoration. Replace the water every couple of days with fresh warm water. Remove any part of the flower which is dying or fading, and cut out dead flowers to allow buds to open out. You could also place a charcoal tablet in the water, to keep it pure.

If arranging roses, make them last longer by snipping off the bottom inch of the stem with a slanting cut as soon as you get the roses home. To make the water uptake easier, split the lower 2 inches of the stem with a knife, or bash it with a hammer. Soak the flowers up to their necks overnight before arranging them, with only the flower heads visible above the water line. The following morning, arrange the flowers in a vase of fresh water, and remember that all flowers will last longer in a cool room.

Flower Arrangements in the Home

If you like to have lots of flowers around your home, do you usually place these only in the lounge or dining areas of your home? Have you ever considered putting flowers in the kitchen area? As with any arrangement, it is important to consider the colour scheme of the room, as well as what you wish to achieve with the arrangement. If you are thinking of having several types of flower, it is important to maintain a central theme. White or cream flowers, such as narcissi, with plenty of sprigs of green foliage will give kitchens a clean, crisp look. As we have already learnt, colour can have a dramatic effect on our senses, and it is important that we decide from the outset whether our decoration is to have impact and make a statement, or whether it should blend in with the existing decor of the room. Tulips always look good when displayed in the correct container, especially when they are allowed to fall naturally. The bright colour of the daffodil or yellow narcissus can enhance a room and bring life into the surroundings. By putting together several bunches of the same colour flowers, you can make a topiary effect or ball shape, especially if you ensure that all the flower heads face outwards. Keeping all the stems parallel to form a sort of trunk, secure them with garden twine or raffia just beneath the flower heads to maintain the shape. Bright colours will give a cheering effect to a room. In the spring, a small jug with tulips, marigolds and catkins or an arrangement of purple and yellow hellebores creates a seasonal theme in your home. When looking for a container for flowers, don't always just reach for the normal vase, however decorative it may be in itself. Try to be a little adventurous and think about milk jugs, sugar bowls, soup tureens and other such containers.

Giving Gifts

We have looked at many aspects of flowers, plants and herbs: their meanings, uses, oils, health remedies and superstitions. You may feel that you need some advice as to which flowers or plants you should give as a special gift. Simply buy what you feel gives the message you want to send to the person concerned. If you feel that you want to help pep someone up, you can try the colour suggestions we discussed earlier. You could make a special arrangement of dried flowers, make your own herbal infusions or make a scented pillow for someone who is ill. However, if you feel that all that is required to make someone realise they are special to you is a nice bouquet of flowers with a well-worded card, why change what has worked before! I have tried to give you lots of information in this book on ways in which flowers, plants and herbs can be and have been used for gifts, for health and beauty care, and for decoration. I have not presumed to try to tell anybody what gifts they should give to people in their lives, nor will 1. It is, after all, the thought that counts and not the gift. You can, however, start to think of colours and the impact they have. You might also now wish to include home-made cosmetics or home-made dried flower arrangements as part of your gift ideas. I feel that home-made gifts mean more because I know that the person concerned has taken the time and trouble not only to think about the gift, but also to make it as well. Making gifts adds to the impact of the gift and will also give you great pleasure to make. If you have family or friends who are ill, why not give a herbal gift? Which colours will help them to feel a little better, which oils might ease their pain or create an uplifting atmosphere?

If you have family or friends who are elderly and have trouble with their gardens you could help them re-plan their garden to get the best from it from both a colour and a health angle. You might be able to persuade them to think about herbal remedies.

Using Flowers in Decoration

Some lucky people seem to have a natural talent for flower decoration. Unfortunately this doesn't apply to many people, myself included. I can make an arrangement look reasonably good, but wouldn't class myself an expert by any stretch of the imagination. The following tips have been picked up from experts. I would suggest that novices, like myself, allow themselves ample time for all the necessary work, so that the decoration isn't rushed. Forward planning is a must; as it is futile leaving the flower decorations intended for a dinner party until ten minutes before your guests are due to arrive. As with gardening, flower arranging can be quite a therapeutic pastime - it can help you to unwind and relax, and it can give a great deal of satisfaction. If you are new to flower decoration, begin with something relatively simple and then work towards more complicated forms and shapes.

Location, Design and Balance

When thinking about your design, consider where it is to be placed. There are many areas around homes which would benefit from a flower arrangement either on a permanent basis or perhaps in the summer months. One such area is a fireplace. Generally speaking, a fireplace is not actively used during the summer months. Flower arrangements designed for the fireplace can completely transform a stagnant area and form a focal point. We don't necessarily have to use a dried flower arrangement. We can use seasonal blooms, vary the shades and predominant colours, and create a different effect from one week to another. We can add colour to our homes with flowers at any time of the year, and as the world market in flowers opens up, we are not limited to flowers native to our home country. Seasonal shades of flowers, fruits and shrubs can greatly enhance a room by imitating the colours of nature. Spring colours can be pastel shades, such as pale lilacs, light blues and pinks, and also the colour of apple blossom or combinations of pale yellows and white. Summer colours include reds, yellows, striking colours, but also the colours of strawberry, apricot and other fruits. Autumn shades, with russets, golds and reds can also add something to a room. Many people think of winter as a colourless time, but one only has to think of the bright red berries of the holly bush, striking red poinsettias and the pure white of the mistletoe and Christmas roses to realise that with a little thought, colour can be brought into the home even at the bleakest of times. Wild flowers, such as the common thistle and gorse, especially at the end of the year when buying flowers might be an expensive hobby, add extra colour when combined with fruit. Fruit can be included in any flower decoration, but remember to replace this when it is obviously past its best. When using flowers to decorate a room, clusters of any colour, even pale colours, can be as central a feature in a design as the most carefully chosen deep-coloured flowers. The size and the placement of the decoration are crucial.

Many homes, especially the older homes built at a time when hallways were central features, may have a hall mirror. Often the mirror is seldom used, and one striking way of using a flower decoration to maximum effect is to place flowers in front of a mirror to reflect both the light and the colour of the flowers. Many homes have an alcove area either side of a chimney breast and to utilise these spaces it is often used for shelving or a table and is often placed in this area. Why not consider inserting lights in the alcoves for illuminating flower decorations. If you are creating a table centrepiece, consider the wood that the table is made of, its colour and its textures.

Before you start any decoration, make sure that you look at the colours already in the room. Often people think of a design, buy some flowers and arrange them in the kitchen area and then find, on transporting them to the place where they are to go, that the colour does not work or the design is too bulky/small/tall for the intended position. For this reason I would suggest that you arrange the flowers in the spot where they are to be displayed. Perhaps the most important consideration when making a flower arrangement is to decide what it is you wish to achieve. Having decided upon this, you must look at colours and at what flowers are available to you. It is important that you like the shape of the flowers, enjoy their fragrance, and ensure that the flowers you decide upon are easily available - look in your garden first, or if you prefer to bring in wildflowers, take a walk in the country and see what is about. If you are making a flower decoration for someone else, take their likes and dislikes into account, and be sensitive over flowers which have memories for the person concerned. If you are going to buy flowers from a florist, bear in mind the cost, especially if finances are limited. Making a quick sketch of what you are intending to do may help you to decide how many flowers you need. You don't have to be an artist, any little sketch will suffice. Think about how the colours blend together, the height of the blooms, and the space you have to fill. Think of design, think of the shape, the height and width you want - don't just think of rounded shapes, with larger blooms and stalks on the outer edges of your arrangement and smaller blooms coming inwards. Think also of triangles, rectangles or even half circles. It is also important to think about symmetry — make sure both sides of your design balance out. You will need some foliage to act as a buffer between two strong colours - this need not necessarily be green. Roses and orchids make a nice combination - as the overall shape and form of the flowers harmonises. You also have to make sure that you don't choose flowers which are ill matched on a scale theme such as gladioli with lilies of the valley. Choose flowers of similar sizes, or place taller flowers at the rear of the design, gradually sloping downwards to smaller blooms.

If you wish to create a design which will help you from a colour angle to relax or unwind, remember what we have learnt about colour and how it affects us. If you want to create a striking arrangement, reds, yellows and oranges work, but don't make the arrangement too startling, especially if your aim is one of creating a relaxing focus. If you want something a little more soothing, think about delicate flowers and blue pinks, mauves, blues and softer tones. Vary the theme with grey or silvery foliage and remember that there are many plants with different shaped leaves which can help to create something more unusual - pointed foliage, such as the leaves of flax, can help to make the arrangement interesting, and dried ears of wheat in an arrangement will work well at any time of the year. You might also consider a blend of different shades of one colour from pale to dark. The problem with just one colour is that you need to create a design which will still make a statement, so try not to place the flowers level with each other, and think about adding a little variety of colour by varying the foliage to add interest. A focal point to your design is what professionals call 'the heart' of the arrangement. This need not necessarily be just one flower – a group of four of five flowers of varying sizes or three flowers surrounded by leaves might be more interesting.

The choice of container for the arrangement is important. Make sure that the colour of the container matches in with your arrangement. Avoid placing large flowers in a container which is too small to balance them. A circular vase or bowl really demands a circular design, and remember that the first placement of flowers must be firm as the rest of the arrangement will be built around it. You may wish to experiment with different containers, such as a copper tea-urn, a large wine glass or other more unusual containers. I have seen very effective arrangements in things as diverse as a vinegar jar and a warming pan. We now have this wonderful stuff called florists' foam, which can be used equally well on its own as it can with a container, and it is very useful in spaces where we might not normally be able to have flowers, such as long and narrow spaces. You don't always want your flower decoration to stick too far into a room or intrude on your guests or family.

Good summer colours are oranges, yellows and blues. White also works well in summertime. Pale colours work well any time, and winter is the time when a splash of red or green will help cheer up the cold winter evenings. Silver and gold also work well in wintertime, and dried flowers, with a few gold- or silver-painted cones and leaves, or seasonal clusters of berries or fruit, will help make a beautiful arrangement. As your flower arrangement is an important part of the room, be sure to have ornaments in your room which complement it.

We all make mistakes when starting out on flower decorations, and even the professionals don't always get it right, so don't be afraid to experiment a little. Review what we have already said about starting a design and perhaps write yourself a little list of pointers.

Hanging baskets are a popular form of arrangement, and will help to bring the garden area a little nearer to the home. Many garden centres will make up a hanging basket for you, and even if you have never tried one before, you might now wish to consider having a hanging basket outside your door or in the porch area, irrespective of the time of year. Even those of us with little or no garden can then benefit from the colours, textures and fragrances of plants and flowers.

If you are hoping to attract a little romance to a dinner party, or create a cosy atmosphere, think of adding candles to your flower centre-piece. Likewise, a few floating candles in a bowl of water near to an arrangement, will add a little extra glow. If you are using candles or night-lights remember to keep them away from the flowers for safety reasons.

Objects for Flower Arrangements

If you are now ready to embark upon making a flower decoration, there are some materials you might wish to get ready. A selection of different kinds of wire is important for arrangements. Stiff wire, for example, is great for dried flower arrangements, and finer wire comes in useful for many fresh arrangements. Pin holders, putty or plasticine, available from most florists can also help keep your arrangement in shape.

Florist's foam is indispensable for any type of arrangement as it can be cut to any shape and size and can be concealed with moss or dried flowers. Most of the wet foam available can be soaked through in a couple of minutes and can be easily taped or wired in place. Most stems, if cut at an angle, will push into florist's foam easily, but if extremely delicate make a hole first with a spike. It is really important to make sure that the florist's foam is kept damp, so top up the container with fresh water regularly, especially in hot conditions.

You could try putting stones or coloured marbles in the bottom of vases to help stabilise arrangements. This also adds to the appearance of the arrangement, especially if the marbles echo the colour of the flowers, and the vase is clear glass. Also available from a variety of outlets are coloured crystals which will take in water, provide colour and keep flower arrangements fresh for a long time. Crystals add colour in a different way, and are especially useful in creating an overall theme. Crystals can also be bought to use with house plants and are said to reduce watering to an absolute minimum, so are quite handy for those of us who fail to remember to water our plants on a regular basis.

This book has not been aimed at making us professional gardeners, nor has it attempted to make us florists, herbalists, aromatherapists or interior design consultants. The aim has been to bring the world of nature a little more to the forefront of our minds, to consider the various health benefits available to us all from within the plant world, and to consider how flowers themselves and their colours can help us to achieve more of a balance within our busy lives. So often people, when considering natural remedies only go as far as herbal remedies and commercially available health products. Many of us fail to appreciate how colours, shapes, fragrances and textures affect us on a daily basis. We may enjoy sitting in a beautiful garden and relaxing without realising the beneficial effect this has on our health and well-being. Even those people who live in flats with no garden area at all can bring the world of plants and colour into their lives and benefit as a result. We can all, irrespective of gender, consider using what is naturally available to us in the plant world to our benefit, perhaps by making our own herbal tisanes, by using herbs or fragrances, by making cosmetics, or by using the power of aroma therapy or colour.

We take so much for granted in this world, and often fail to appreciate what we have at our disposal. We seem so intent on making ourselves comfortable and spending time on our material lives that we fail to appreciate our surroundings. Many years ago, I was in hospital with a serious illness and I remember standing at the hospital window and feeling the wind hit my face, and vowing that I would never take such things for granted again. Perhaps we should all stop from time to time and look at the world of nature and remember how privileged we are to have it there.

I hope that some of the information given within this book will do just that, and that you may now enjoy better health and wellbeing by using the power of plants.

Made in the USA
San Bernardino, CA
05 January 2017